Manual of Infection Control in Orthopedic Surgery

Operation Theater Protocols and Patient Optimization

Manual of Infection Control in Orthopedic Surgery

Operation Theater Protocols and Patient Optimization

Second Edition

Parag Kantilal Sancheti FRCS (Ed) MS (ortho) DNB (ortho) MCh (UK)
Professor and Chairman
Sancheti Institute for Orthopaedics and Rehabilitation
Pune, Maharashtra, India

Ashok Shyam MS (ortho)
Orthopedic Surgeon and Research Consultant
Sancheti Institute for Orthopaedics and Rehabilitation
Pune, Maharashtra, India

Foreword
Javad Parvizi MD FRCS

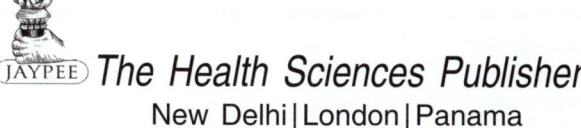

The Health Sciences Publisher
New Delhi | London | Panama

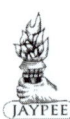

Jaypee Brothers Medical Publishers (P) Ltd

Headquarters
Jaypee Brothers Medical Publishers (P) Ltd.
4838/24, Ansari Road, Daryaganj
New Delhi 110 002, India
Phone: +91-11-43574357
Fax: +91-11-43574314
Email: jaypee@jaypeebrothers.com

Overseas Offices

J.P. Medical Ltd
83 Victoria Street, London
SW1H 0HW (UK)
Phone: +44 20 3170 8910
Fax: +44 (0)20 3008 6180
Email: info@jpmedpub.com

Jaypee-Highlights Medical Publishers Inc
City of Knowledge, Bld. 235, 2nd Floor, Clayton
Panama City, Panama
Phone: +1 507-301-0496
Fax: +1 507-301-0499
Email: cservice@jphmedical.com

Jaypee Brothers Medical Publishers (P) Ltd
17/1-B Babar Road, Block-B, Shaymali
Mohammadpur, Dhaka-1207, Bangladesh
Mobile: +08801912003485
Email: jaypeedhaka@gmail.com

Jaypee Brothers Medical Publishers (P) Ltd
Bhotahity, Kathmandu, Nepal
Phone +977-9741283608
Email: kathmandu@jaypeebrothers.com

Website: www.jaypeebrothers.com
Website: www.jaypeedigital.com

© 2017, Jaypee Brothers Medical Publishers

The views and opinions expressed in this book are solely those of the original contributor(s)/author(s) and do not necessarily represent those of editor(s) of the book.

All rights reserved. No part of this publication may be reproduced, stored or transmitted in any form or by any means, electronic, mechanical, photocopying, recording or otherwise, without the prior permission in writing of the publishers.

All brand names and product names used in this book are trade names, service marks, trademarks or registered trademarks of their respective owners. The publisher is not associated with any product or vendor mentioned in this book.

Medical knowledge and practice change constantly. This book is designed to provide accurate, authoritative information about the subject matter in question. However, readers are advised to check the most current information available on procedures included and check information from the manufacturer of each product to be administered, to verify the recommended dose, formula, method and duration of administration, adverse effects and contraindications. It is the responsibility of the practitioner to take all appropriate safety precautions. Neither the publisher nor the author(s)/editor(s) assume any liability for any injury and/or damage to persons or property arising from or related to use of material in this book.

This book is sold on the understanding that the publisher is not engaged in providing professional medical services. If such advice or services are required, the services of a competent medical professional should be sought.

Every effort has been made where necessary to contact holders of copyright to obtain permission to reproduce copyright material. If any have been inadvertently overlooked, the publisher will be pleased to make the necessary arrangements at the first opportunity.

Inquiries for bulk sales may be solicited at: jaypee@jaypeebrothers.com

Manual of Infection Control in Orthopedic Surgery: Operation Theater Protocols and Patient Optimization

First Edition: 2015
Second Edition: **2017**
ISBN: 978-93-85999-30-7

Printed at Rajkamal Electric Press, Plot No. 2, Phase-IV, Kundli, Haryana.

Dedicated
to

Our Patients
Who have motivated us to work for improvement of healthcare standards

Our Parents
Their endless love and support has been a constant source of inspiration to us

Mentors

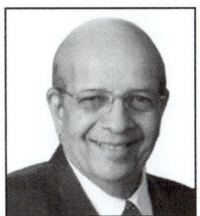

KH Sancheti FRCS (Edinburgh) MS PhD (Ortho)
Founder President
Sancheti Institute for Orthopaedics and Rehabilitation
Pune, Maharashtra, India

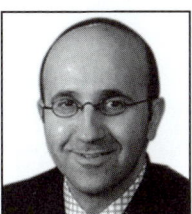

Javad Parvizi MD FRCS
Professor of Orthopedic Surgery
Rothman Institute at Thomas
Jefferson University Hospital
Philadelphia, USA

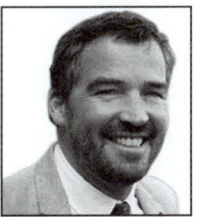

Olivier Borens MD PhD
*Head of the Department of Septic Surgery and
Head of the Orthopedic-trauma Unit of the
Department for the Musculoskeletal System*
University Hospital in Lausanne
Lausanne, Switzerland

Contributors

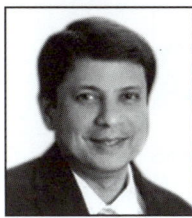

Editor
Parag Kantilal Sancheti
FRCS (Ed), MS (ortho), DNB (ortho), MCh (UK)
Professor & Chairman
Sancheti Institute for Orthopaedics and Rehabilitation
Pune, Maharashtra, India

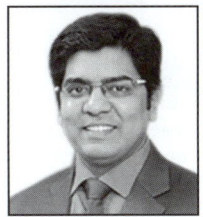

Editor
Ashok Shyam MS (Ortho)
Orthopedic Surgeon and Research Consultant
Sancheti Institute for Orthopaedics and Rehabilitation
Pune, Maharashtra, India

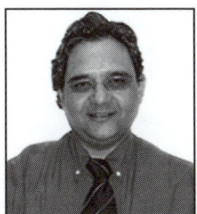

Editor
Rajeev Joshi MS (Ortho)
Professor and Orthopedic Surgeon
Sancheti Institute for Orthopaedics and Rehabilitation
Pune, Maharashtra, India

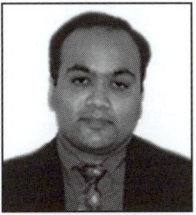

Editor
Steve Rocha MCh (Ortho) FAGE (MAN)
Hand and Microvascular Surgeon
Sancheti Institute for Orthopaedics and Rehabilitation
Pune, Maharashtra, India

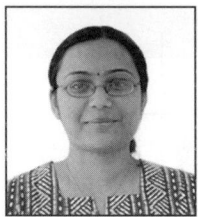

Aditi Malpani MBBS DNB Medicine
Consultant Physician
Sancheti Institute for Orthopaedics
and Rehabilitation
Pune, Maharashtra, India

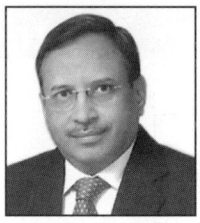

Anil Jain MS MAMS
Professor of Orthopedics
University College of Medical Sciences
University of Delhi
Delhi, India

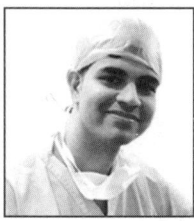

Ali J Electricwala MS (Ortho) DNB
Consultant in Orthopedics and Lecturer
Sancheti Institute for Orthopaedics
and Rehabilitation
Pune, Maharashtra, India

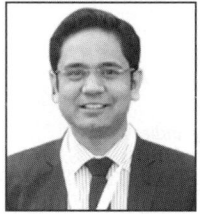

Amol Narkhede MS (Ortho)
Consultant Trauma Surgeon
Sancheti Institute for Orthopaedics
and Rehabilitation
Pune, Maharashtra, India

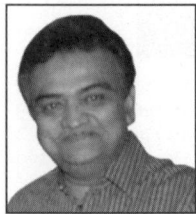

Bharat S Mody MCh (Ortho)
ODTS (RCSE)
Director and Chief Arthroplasty Surgeon
Welcare Hospital
Vadodara, Gujarat, India

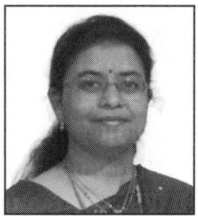

Bharati Adhye MD (Anesthesiology)
Chief Consultant Anesthesiologist
Sancheti Institute for Orthopaedics
and Rehabilitation
Pune, Maharashtra, India

Contributors

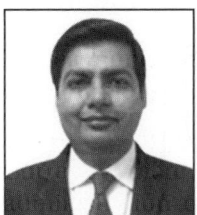

Chetan Oswal MS (Ortho)
Orthopedic Consultant
Sancheti Institute for Orthopaedics
and Rehabilitation
Pune, Maharashtra, India

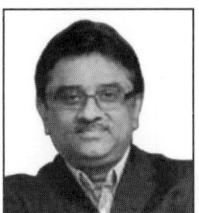

Gurava Reddy D (Ortho) DNB (Ortho)
MCh FRCS
Chairman and Chief Joint Replacement Surgeon
Sunshine Bone and Joint Institute
Hyderabad, Andhra Pradesh, India

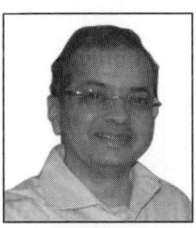

Hemant M Wakankar MS (Ortho)
DNB FRCS MCh
Specialist in Joint Replacement Surgery
Deenanath Mangeshkar Hospital
and Ruby Hall Clinic
Pune, Maharashtra, India

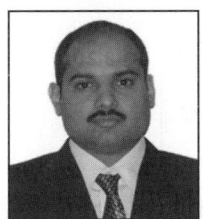

Himanshu Dongre MD (Anesthesiology)
Consultant Anesthesiologist
Sancheti Institute for Orthopaedics
and Rehabilitation
Pune, Maharashtra, India

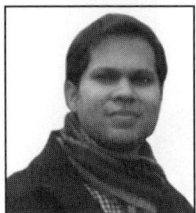

Lovey Singhal MS (Ortho)
MCh (Dundee)
Consultant in Orthopedics
Sancheti Institute for Orthopaedics
and Rehabilitation
Pune, Maharashtra, India

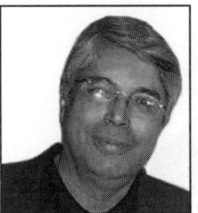

Madhav Borate MS (Ortho)
Director, Department of Orthopedics
Samarth Hospital
Pune, Maharashtra, India

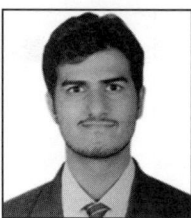

Mayur P Kardile MS (Ortho) DNB
Fellow in Spine Surgery
Sancheti Institute for Orthopaedics
and Rehabilitation
Pune, Maharashtra, India

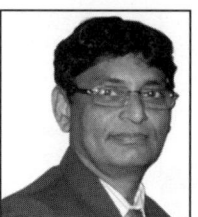

Pramod P Neema DNB (Ortho) FICA
Director and Consultant Joint Replacement Surgeon
Unique Super Specialty Hospital
Indore, Maharashtra, India

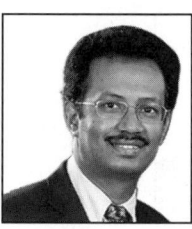

Rajasekaran S FRCS MCh FACS
Chairman
Ganga Hospital
Coimbatore, Tamil Nadu, India

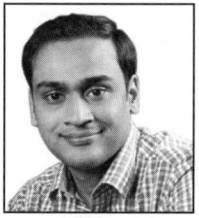

Sachin Jain MS (Ortho) DNB (Ortho)
Lecturer and Fellow in Arthroscopy
Ganga Hospital
Coimbatore, Tamil Nadu, India

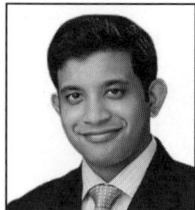

Vivek Vincent Valiyaveettil MS (Ortho)
Consultant
Sancheti Institute for Orthopaedics
and Rehabilitation
Pune, Maharashtra, India

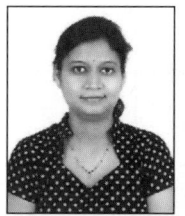

Vaishali Tadokar MD
(Medical Microbiology)
Consultant
Infection Control and Microbiology
Sancheti Institute of Orthopaedics
and Rehabilitation
Pune, Maharashtra, India

Foreword

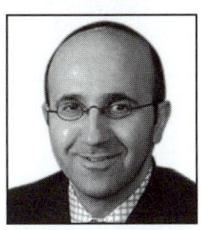

Infection is a devastating complication of surgical procedures. Periprosthetic joint infection (PJI) results in a terrible outcome of an otherwise successful surgical procedure, including significantly increased mortality. Recent studies have shown that patients developing PJI have worse 'survivorship', than patients with cancer. What is amazingly disappointing is that despite all efforts, the incidence of PJI has not changed over the last three to four decades. It is heartwarming to note that the medical community has taken the issue of infection seriously and is collectively orchestrating efforts to prevent this devastating complication. The center for disease control is in the final throw of publishing their surgical site infection (SSI) prevention guidelines. The World Health Organization (WHO) has just begun a similar effort to determine the strategies that can result in reduction of the SSI. In August 2013, an International Consensus Group convened 400 experts from 50 countries to establish best practice guides. These are some examples of the efforts in recent years that are attempting to strike at the heart of the issue in hand.

The book *Manual of Infection Control in Orthopedic Surgery: Operation Theater Protocols and Patient Optimization* is an example of elegant efforts that are invested to determine measures that can be effective in reducing infection after orthopedic procedures. The editors, Parag Sancheti, Rajeev Joshi, Ashok Shyam and Steve Rocha have produced a body of literature that is likely to be used by many, for the years to come. Congratulations to the editors and authors for producing this great masterpiece.

Javad Parvizi MD FRCS
Professor of Orthopedic Surgery
Rothman Institute at Thomas Jefferson University Hospital
Philadelphia, USA

Preface to the Second Edition

Welcome to the second edition of the book *Manual of Infection Control in Orthopedic Surgery: Operation Theater Protocols and Patient Optimization*. The impact of the first edition was widely felt in the surgical community and it encouraged us to write the second edition of the book. Healthcare-associated infections or infections acquired in healthcare settings are 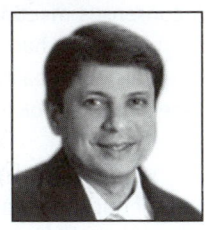 the most frequent adverse events in healthcare delivery worldwide. Hundreds of millions of patients are affected by healthcare-associated infections worldwide each year, leading to significant mortality and financial losses for health systems.

World Health Organization (WHO) statistics have revealed that for every 100 hospitalized patients at any given time, 7 in developed and 10 in developing countries will acquire at least one healthcare-associated infection. In developing countries, financial constraints may inhibit acquisition of state-of-the-art equipment to prevent infection. Yet, the need for such nursing homes is evident from the fact that in developing country like India, recent statistics have revealed that the ratio of doctors to patients is 1:1,619.

The International Consensus Meeting for infection control in total knee replacement surgery held in Philadelphia under the auspices of Dr Javad Parvizi was an eye-opener for us to study, how we could control infection in orthopedic surgeries in developing countries like India. We are, however, diversified into studying the infection in not just arthroplasty, but trauma and spine as well. Holding the pattern similar to the first edition, we set out by discussing the various reasons that cause infection in the pre-, peri and intra-operative settings. We held meetings every week for almost a year and our team gradually grew with consultants volunteering to research different aspects of possible causes of infection. With an emphasis on evidence-based medicine, we reviewed literature and where there were deficiencies, we relied on different opinions of stalwarts in the field of orthopedics. A consensus meeting was held wherein doctors from all over India, most of whom had tremendous experience in setting up their own hospitals and dealing with infections, were invited to review every aspect of the book and share their experience and knowledge on the same.

We developed guidelines keeping in mind the problems faced by smaller nursing homes with regards to space constraints and financial limitations. With a question-and answer-based approach, we tried to make this book *Manual of Infection Control in Orthopedic Surgery: Operation Theater Protocols and Patient Optimization*, easy to read and simple to understand. We included common questions asked and tried to make the answers more applicable to conditions in nursing homes and smaller hospitals, which plays an important role in the healthcare delivery system in developing countries.

We were honored to be under the guidance of Dr KH Sancheti, Founder President of Sancheti Hospital. Dr Olivier Borens also reviewed our proceedings and his inputs were a constant source of inspiration for us to complete this endeavor. We had a lot of inputs from Dr Bharat S Mody, Dr Hemant M Wakankar and Dr Pramod P Neema and many others whose contributions have made this book what it is today.

We hope this book will guide orthopedic surgeons who are venturing to start their own hospitals. It would be a boon for postgraduates with simple answers to commonly asked questions as well. It would be an immense resource for anyone to understand and prevent infections in orthopedic practice.

Parag K Sancheti

Preface to the First Edition

Healthcare-associated infections or infections acquired in healthcare settings are the most frequent adverse events in healthcare delivery worldwide. Hundreds of millions of patients are affected by healthcare-associated infections worldwide each year, leading to significant mortality and financial losses for health systems.

World Health Organization statistics have revealed that for every 100 hospitalized patients at any given time, 7 in developed and 10 in developing countries will acquire at least one healthcare-associated infection. In developing countries, financial constraints may inhibit acquisition of state-of-the-art equipment to prevent infection. Yet, the need for such nursing homes is evident from the fact that in developing country like India, recent statistics have revealed that the ratio of doctors to patients is 1:1,619.

The International Consensus Meeting for infection control in total knee replacement surgery held in Philadelphia under the auspices of Dr Javad Parvizi was an eye-opener for us to study, how we could control infection in orthopedic surgeries in developing countries like India. We are, however, diversified into studying the infection in not just arthroplasty, but trauma and spine as well. We set out by discussing the various reasons that cause infection in the pre-, peri- and intra-operative settings. We held meetings every week for almost a year and our team gradually grew with consultants volunteering to research different aspects of possible causes of infection. With an emphasis on evidence-based medicine, we reviewed literature and where there were deficiencies, we relied on different opinions of stalwarts in the field of orthopedics. A consensus meeting was held wherein doctors from all over India, most of whom had tremendous experience in setting up their own hospitals, were invited to review each aspect and share their experience and knowledge on the same. We developed guidelines keeping in mind the problems faced by smaller nursing homes with regards to space constraints and financial limitations.

With a question-and answer-based approach, we tried to make this book *'Manual of Infection Control in Orthopedic Surgery Operation Theater Protocols and Patient Optimization'* easy to read and simple to understand. We included common questions asked and tried to make the answers more applicable to conditions in nursing homes and smaller hospitals, which plays an important role in the healthcare delivery system in developing countries.

We were honored to be under the guidance of Dr KH Sancheti, Founder President of Sancheti Hospital. Dr Olivier Borens also reviewed our proceedings and his inputs were a constant source of inspiration for us to complete this endeavor. We had a lot of inputs from Dr Bharat Mody, Dr Hemant Wakankar and Dr Pramod Neema and many others whose contributions has made this book what it is today.

We hope this book will guide orthopedic surgeons who are venturing to start their own hospitals. It would be a boon for postgraduates with simple answers to commonly asked questions as well. It should be an immense resource for anyone to understand and prevent infection in orthopedic practice.

Parag K Sancheti

Acknowledgments

This project is an initiative of Sancheti Research Department. The idea of this project was conceived from the 'proceedings of the International Consensus Meeting on Periprosthetic Joint Infection' and we would like to thank Dr Javad Parvizi for inspiring us in writing this book.

We also received support from the Indian Orthopaedic Research Group and its members, and we thank them for their time and effort.

Special thanks to Dr Ravishek Kumar for taking time out to attend our weekly meetings from the start of the project and for his valuable inputs during discussion.

We thank Dr Olivier Borens for visiting us and spending time to go through the entire document and giving his constructive suggestions.

Sancheti Research Department needs a special mention. A project is always an amalgamation of knowledge, expertize, guidance, leadership and support from the team. Special thanks to Neelam Jhanjiani and the rest of the research department, Nalini Gawande, Chaitali Deshmukh, Nutan Jadhav and Archana Gawali for their support.

I gratefully acknowledge the help of Shri Jitendar P Vij (Group Chairman), Mr Ankit Vij (Group President), Ms Chetna Malhotra Vohra (Associate Director–Content Strategy) and Ms Payal Bharti (Project Manager) Jaypee Brothers Medical Publishers (P) Ltd, New Delhi for their all-round support as and when needed.

Parag K Sancheti
Ashok Shyam

Contents

Section 1: Operation Theater Norms and Protocols

1. Sterilization 3
   Vaishali Tadokar, Bharat S Mody, Hemant M Wakankar

2. Operation Theater Planning and Protocols 17
   Sancheti KH, Ali J Electricwala, Bharat S Mody, Rajasekaran S

   Epoxy Coating of Floors 24
   Vinyl/Linoleum Flooring 25
   Electrogalvanized Powder Coated Sheets 25
   High Pressure Laminates 25
   Suitable Materials for Floor Coatings 26
   Bacillocid Rasant 28

3. Surgeon Preparation and Scrubbing Protocols 31
   Vivek Vincent Valiyaveettil, Gurava Reddy, Ashok Shyam,
   Parag K Sancheti

4. Laminar Airflow and Air-handling Unit 37
   Sancheti KH, Ali J Electricwala, Rajasekaran S, Bharat S Mody

   Laminar Airflow in the Operating Room 38

5. Operation Theater Personnel 46
   Lovey Singhal, Steve Rocha, Rajeev Joshi, Madhav Borate

Section 2: Perioperative Patient Preparation

6. Patient Optimization 55
   Aditi Malpani, Himanshu Dongre, Bharati Adhye,
   Pramod P Neema, Ashok Shyam

7. Patient and Operative Site Preparation 84
   Madhav Borate, Hemant M Wakankar

8. Intraoperative Protocols 95
   Amol Narkhede, Anil Jain, Parag K Sancheti, Hemant M Wakankar

9. Postoperative Management 107
   Chetan Oswal, Sachin Jain, Steve Rocha, Ashok Shyam, Anil Jain

10. Prophylactic Antibiotics 124
    Mayur P Kardile, Chetan Oswal, Ashok Shyam, Parag Sancheti

Further Reading 133

Editorial

We welcome our readers to the second edition of the book.

Surgical site infections (SSIs) are one of the most devastating complications in orthopedic surgery and has a huge impact in terms of healthcare burden and patient morbidity. However, SSIs are something that can be prevented to a large extent. The two most important factors that can be optimized for prevention of SSIs are—operation theater protocols and surgical optimization. Again these two factors vary depending on the geography and socioeconomic status, especially in a country like India. Thus, even though few guidelines are available from world bodies, these are mostly applicable to the Western World. There is a need to adapt and modify these guidelines to fit the needs of Indian surgical scenario. Also, there are certain aspects like privately owned nursing homes and small collaborative hospital, which present unique circumstances for developing an infection control guideline. The patient profile in our country is very varied, requiring new methods to approach their issues. Moreover, orthopedic surgery as a faculty has grown in leaps and bounds in the last decade with new technological advancements and innovations, which still require customization to our scenario. Lastly, during the course of development of this project we realized that literature is lacking on many points and when available are applicable to either the Western World or to a very narrow band of situations. In these situations, it was necessary to call in expert opinions, which would allow us to reach a rational consensus. Throughout this book we have followed the similar pattern with literature review combined with expert consensus to come up with the logical conclusions, which are applicable to varying scenario. For the same reason we decided to present the book in a question-answer format so that specific points from literature and consensus can be highlighted.

Keeping in mind all these factors and specially the Indian circumstances, this group for setting up the infection control guidelines was formed under the leadership of Dr Parag Sancheti. More than 30 orthopedic consultants have contributed into making this manuscript and a period of more than 10 months has been invested in preparing this manual. Regular weekly meeting culminated in a final full day 'Consensus' meet in Pune where all the questions were discussed with the experts from across the country. Also the experts from allied fields like microbiology, anesthesia and internal medicine also contributed in this proceedings. This book is compiled in two separate sections namely: ***Section 1:*** Operation Theater Norms and Protocols and ***Section 2:*** Perioperative Patient Preparation. Each section has 5 chapters with a team of experts working on each subgroups taking into consideration the relevant literature and also consulting the experts on the topics to get their opinions.

Section 1: Operation Theater Norms and Protocols

Includes Following Chapters

Chapter 1: Sterilization

This subgroup focuses on the sterilization methods and protocols in general and then goes on to answer specific questions like sterilization of instruments, implants, linen, monitoring of the sterilization process and some points on CSSD functioning.

Chapter 2: Operation Theater Planning and Protocols

This is one of the most important chapter of the book and includes detailed review of OT planning and it would be very helpful for surgeons planning to build a new hospital or even for upgrading the existing facility. Indian scenario and requirements are taken into consideration while writing this chapter.

Chapter 3: Surgeon Preparation and Scrubbing Protocols

Lot of variability has been noted in these protocols and huge amount of literature was consulted before putting together this chapter. The protocols are simplified and practical.

Chapter 4: Laminar Airflow and Air-handling Unit

This topic is one of the widely discussed topics especially in context to orthopedic OT complexes. A simplified explanation of the air-handling unit (AHU) and practical guidelines for implementation of a good AHU is provided in this chapter.

Chapter 5: Operation Theater Personnel

Operation Theater personnel play a very important role in functioning of an optimal OT complex. This chapter focusses on their conduct and also provides guidelines related to recovery rooms.

Section 2: Perioperative Patient Preparation

Includes Following Chapters

Chapter 6: Patient Optimization

This is one of the most extensively reviewed chapters in this book and we have tried to provide only relevant and practical points covering most of the comorbidities and also nutritional status and other optimization parameters.

Chapter 7: Patient and Operative Site Preparation

This chapter focuses on issues like hair removal, scrubbing protocols and draping materials. Standardized guidelines are put for each of these questions.

Chapter 8: Intraoperative Protocols

Intraoperative factors like incise drapes, skin knives, suction tips and irrigation solutions are discussed in this chapter.

Chapter 9: Postoperative Management

Discussion related to wound dressing, wound check and drain protocols are discussed here. Also brief review of a persistently draining wound is provided here.

Chapter 10: Prophylactic Antibiotics

Detailed protocol of antibiotics in perioperative period is described here. Special note of antibiotic allergy testing and antibiotic resistance is also included in this section.

Although all these workgroups have been thoroughly researched, we do not claim to be exhaustive. The manual was created with aim to suit the needs of Indian scenario and hence, as far as possible only questions relevant to Indian scenario are included in the book. There are other areas the book would like to include in the next edition but that will depend on the reviews and comments from our readers. We hope this book will serve as a guideline for operation theater standardization and surgical optimization, ultimately reaching the goal of reducing and preventing SSIs. We also hope that this manual will also trigger development of more questions and participation of more surgeons across the country so that we can identify more issues and try and reach a rational consensus for the same or initiate research protocols to answer them.

In the present form, most of our guidelines have considered the elective and emergency case scenarios and have appropriate recommendations. Extensive literature support is provided wherever needed by taking the Indian perspective into account. The unique part of this book is that, it has been written in a simple question answer format, which is very comprehensible.

We believe this to be a exclusive endeavor especially in Indian scenario and we hope many surgeons, hospitals and patients will benefit from this manual.

Parag K Sancheti
Ashok Shyam

Section 1

Operation Theater Norms and Protocols

Section Outline

1. Sterilization
2. Operation Theater Planning and Protocols
3. Surgeon Preparation and Scrubbing Protocols
4. Laminar Airflow and Air-handling Unit
5. Operation Theater Personnel

Sterilization

Vaishali Tadokar, Bharat S Mody, Hemant M Wakankar

INTRODUCTION

Sterilization is essential for ensuring that medical and surgical instruments do not transmit infectious pathogens to patients. Since, sterilization of all patient-care items is not necessary; healthcare policies must identify primarily on the basis of the items intended to be used, whether cleaning, disinfection or sterilization is indicated.

Sterilization describes a process that destroys or eliminates all forms of microbial life and is carried out in healthcare facilities by physical or chemical methods.

Disinfection describes a process that eliminates many or all pathogenic microorganisms, except bacterial spores, on inanimate objects.

Chemical sterilants are disinfectants that kill spores with prolonged exposure times (3–12 hours).

High-level disinfectants are disinfectants that work at similar concentrations, but with shorter exposure periods (e.g. 20 minutes for 2% glutaraldehyde) will kill all microorganisms except large numbers of bacterial spores.

Low-level disinfectants can kill most vegetative bacteria, some fungi and some viruses in a practical period of time (< 10 minutes).

Intermediate-level disinfectants might be cidal for mycobacteria, vegetative bacteria, most viruses and most fungi, but do not necessarily kill bacterial spores.

What is the most common method of sterilization used in orthopedic setup?

- **Steam** sterilizer is the most common method used for sterilization of instruments and linen as it is nontoxic, inexpensive, rapidly microbicidal and sporicidal.
- The pre vacuum type of steam sterilizer is most commonly used.

Explanation[1]

Sterilization is a process that destroys or eliminates all forms of microbial life and is carried out in healthcare facilities by physical or chemical methods.

Sterilization methods include:
- High temperature sterilization:
  - Steam sterilization
  - Flash sterilization
  - Dry heat sterilization.

Description

High Temperature Sterilization
- **Steam sterilization:** It is nontoxic, inexpensive, rapidly microbicidal and sporicidal. Steam sterilization, as accomplished in an autoclave, is to expose each item to direct steam contact at the required temperature and pressure for the specified time. Moist heat in the form of saturated steam under pressure is the most widely used and the most dependable.
  - **Gravity type:** 30 minutes at 121°C (250°F) in a gravity displacement.
  - **Pre vacuum type:** 4 minutes at 132°C (270°F) in a pre vacuum sterilizer.
  - **Steam-flush pressure-pulsing process:** It is a process, which removes air rapidly by repeatedly alternating a steam flush and a pressure pulse above atmospheric pressure.

- **Flash sterilization:** Sterilization of an unwrapped object at 132°C for 3 minutes at 27–28 lb of pressure in a gravity displacement sterilizer.
- **Dry heat sterilization:** This method should be used only for materials that might be damaged by moist heat or that are impenetrable to moist heat (e.g. powders, petroleum products, sharp instruments). The primary lethal process is considered to be oxidation of cell constituents.

Advantage

Steam sterilization is nontoxic, relatively low costs, penetrates materials, noncorrosive.

Disadvantage

Slow rate of heat penetration.

What is the use of ethylene oxide and plasma sterilizers in orthopedic setup?

Ethylene oxide (ETO) sterilization and hydrogen peroxide (H_2O_2) gas plasma sterilization has been the most commonly used process for sterilizing temperature and moisture-sensitive medical devices and supplies in healthcare institutions such as arthroscopy instruments, camera head and cables, fiber optic light cables, shaver handpieces, Stryker drill and saw system, endoscopes, corrosion-susceptible metal alloys.

Explanation[1]

Low Temperature Sterilization
- **Ethylene oxide sterilization:** Two types—mixed gas and 100% ETO. ETO is a colorless gas that is flammable and explosive. The four essential parameters are gas concentration (450–1,200 mg/L), temperature (37–63°C), relative humidity (40–80%) (water molecules carry ETO to reactive sites) and exposure time (1–6 hours).

- **Hydrogen peroxide gas plasma sterilization:** Gas plasmas have been referred to as the fourth state of matter (i.e. liquids, solids, gases and gas plasmas). Gas plasmas are generated in an enclosed chamber under deep vacuum using radiofrequency or microwave energy to excite the gas molecules and produce charged particles in the form of free radicals. A free radical is an atom with an unpaired electron and is a highly reactive species that are capable of interacting with essential cell components (e.g. enzymes and nucleic acids) and thereby disrupt the metabolism of microorganisms. The type of seed gas used and the depth of the vacuum are two important variables that can determine the effectiveness of this process.
- **Peracetic acid sterilization:** Peracetic acid is a highly biocidal oxidizer that maintains its efficacy in the presence of organic soil. The diluted peracetic acid is circulated within the chamber of the machine and pumped through the channels of the endoscope for 12 minutes, decontaminating exterior surfaces, lumens and accessories.
- **Ozone sterilization:** Ozone is produced, when O_2 is energized and split into two monatomic (O_1) molecules. The monatomic oxygen molecules then collide with O_2 molecules to form ozone, which is O_3. This additional oxygen atom makes ozone a powerful oxidant that destroys microorganisms, but is highly unstable.
- **Formaldehyde sterilization:** The process involves the use of formalin, which is vaporized into a formaldehyde gas that is admitted into the sterilization chamber.
- **Ionizing radiations:** Sterilization by ionizing radiation, primarily by cobalt 60, gamma rays or electron accelerators, is a low-temperature sterilization method that has been used for a number of medical products (e.g. tissue for transplantation, pharmaceuticals and medical

devices). There are no Food and Drug Administration (FDA) cleared ionizing radiation sterilization processes for use in healthcare facilities.

What is the use of flash/immediate-use steam sterilizer (IUSS) in orthopedic setup?

Flash sterilizer is not recommended to be used for sterilization of instruments.

Explanation[1]

Flash Sterilization

Flash sterilization is a modification of conventional steam sterilization (either gravity, pre vacuum or steam-flush pressure-pulse) in which the flashed item is placed in an open tray or rigid container to allow for rapid penetration of steam. It is not recommended because of the lack of timely biological indicators to monitor performance, absence of protective packaging following sterilization, possibility for contamination of processed items during transportation to the operating rooms and the sterilization cycle parameters (i.e. time, temperature and pressure) are minimal. Implants should never be flash sterilized.

How are the instruments and linen sterilized?

Instruments/linen before sterilization need to go through the process of:

- Decontamination: Manual or mechanical cleaning in water with detergents/enzymatic cleansers
- Packaging: After visual inspection of cleaned and dried instruments, they must be wrapped in ideal sterilization wrap or placed in rigid containers and kept in instrument trays/baskets
- Sterilization: High temperature/low temperature sterilization depending upon the instruments
- Sterile storage room.

Explanation[1,2]

A controlled environment is intended to facilitate effective decontamination, assembly, sterilization and storage, and to minimize environmental contamination and maintain sterility of sterilized items. The Central Sterile Supply Department (CSSD) ideally should be divided into at least three areas:
- Decontamination
- Packaging
- Sterilization and sterile storage room.

Decontamination Area
Instruments must be cleaned using:
- Water with detergents: Water to be used for cleaning should be soft water or preferably demineralized water to protect the instruments from hard ion deposits.
- Stainless steel sinks with air pressure guns and water sprayer, and showers to be available for cannulated instruments.
- Enzymatic cleaners: They are of proteases/lipases/amylases working at neutral/near neutral pH. Dilution, time of contact should be followed according to manufacturer's instruction:
  - Manual cleaning: There are two essential components, friction and fluidics. Friction (e.g. rubbing/scrubbing the soiled area with a brush) is an old and dependable method. Fluidics (i.e. fluids under pressure) is used to remove surgical debris from internal channels after brushing and when the design does not allow passage of a brush through a channel.
  - Mechanical cleaning machines:
    - Ultrasonic cleaner
    - Washer-disinfector.

Ultrasonic Cleaning
Ultrasonic cleaning is mainly recommended for cannulated instruments and others with crevices (hinges and serrations).
Mechanism: Ultrasonic cleaning removes soil by cavitation and implosion in which waves of acoustic energy are propagated in aqueous solutions to disrupt the bonds that hold particulate matter to surfaces.

Packaging
Once instruments are cleaned, dried and inspected, they must be double wrapped or placed in rigid containers and should be arranged in instrument trays/baskets.

An ideal sterilization wrap would successfully address barrier effectiveness, penetrability (i.e. allows sterilant to penetrate), aeration (e.g. allows ETO to dissipate), ease of use, drapeability, flexibility, puncture resistance, tear strength, toxicity, odor, waste disposal, linting, cost and transparency. There are many packing systems:[2]

- **Woven fabrics:** 100% cotton, cotton-polyester blends, synthetic blends
- **Non-woven materials:** Plastic polymers, cellulose fibers, paper pulp
- **Peel pouches:** Plastic/paper, cellophane, polyethylene
- **Rigid containers:** Plastic/metal.

Loading
All items to be sterilized should be arranged, so all surfaces will be directly exposed to the sterilizing agent.

There are several important basic principles for loading a sterilizer:
- Allow for proper sterilant circulation
- Perforated trays should be placed, so the tray is parallel to the shelf
- Non-perforated containers should be placed on their edge (e.g. basins)
- Small items should be loosely placed in wire baskets

- Peel packs should be placed on edge in perforated or mesh bottom racks or baskets.

Storage

Heat sealed, plastic peel-down pouches and wrapped packs sealed in 3 mL (3/1,000 inch) polyethylene; overwrap have been reported to be sterile for as long as 9 months after sterilization.

Sterile supplies should be stored far enough from the floor (8–10 inch), the ceiling (5 inch) and the outside walls (2 inch) to allow for adequate air circulation, ease of cleaning and compliance with local fire codes.

How are the instruments/implants packed before sterilization?

Packing material used for wrapping of instruments depends upon the technique of sterilization (steam/ETO/plasma) and manufacturer's instruction:
- Steam sterilization: Woven/non-woven textile wraps, spunbond/meltblown/spunbond (SMS) wraps, paper–plastic peel pouches.
- Ethylene oxide sterilization: Polyethylene plastic bags, peel pouches of paper/polyethylene polyester laminate, paper/polypropylene polyester laminate.
- Plasma sterilization: Polypropylene wrap, polyolefin-plastic combination (Tyvek) pouches.

The shelf life of linen packing material is approximately 5–10 days.

The shelf life of paper-plastic peel pouches is approximately 3–6 months.

The shelf life of the packing material is event related and is valuable only when the appropriate storage conditions are maintained like humidity, temperature, dust-free environment and if there is no tear/holes in the packaging material.

Explanation[3]

- Personnel should understand how the sterilization method and the items being sterilized affect the selection of the appropriate packaging method and how the packaging method affects sterilization parameters.
- While selecting a packaging system, personnel should obtain and keep on file the manufacturer's test data, instructions for use and care and handling instructions.

An effective packaging material for steam sterilization processing, as a minimum should:

- Allow adequate air removal from steam penetration of the package contents
- Provide an adequate barrier to microorganisms or their vehicles
- Resist tearing or puncture
- Allow a method of sealing that result in a complete seal that is tamper-evident and provides seal
- Integrity
- Be free of toxic ingredients and non-fast dyes
- Be nonlinting
- Cost-effective.

What are the factors affecting the efficacy of cleaning, disinfection and sterilization?

Factors that affect the efficacy of the sterilization.[1]

Table 1.1: Factors affecting sterilization processes

Factors	Effects
Cleaning	Failure to adequately clean instrument results in higher bioburden, protein load and salt concentration
Bioburden	The natural bioburden of used surgical devices is 10^2–10^3 organisms (primarily vegetative bacteria), which is substantially below the 10^5–10^6 spores used with biological indicators

Contd...

Contd…

Factors	Effects
Pathogen type	Spore-forming organisms are most resistant to sterilization and are the test organisms required for Food and Drug Administration (FDA) clearance However, the contaminating microflora on used surgical instruments consists mainly of vegetative bacteria
Protein	Residual protein decreases efficacy of sterilization
Salt	Residual salt decreases efficacy of sterilization much more than the protein load
Biofilm accumulation	Biofilm accumulation reduces efficacy of sterilization by impairing exposure of the sterilant to the microbial cell
Lumen length	Increasing lumen length impairs sterilant penetration
Lumen diameter	Decreasing lumen diameter impairs sterilant penetration
Restricted flow	Device designs that prevent or inhibit this contact (e.g. sharp bends, blind lumens) will decrease sterilization efficacy
Device design and construction	Materials used in construction may affect compatibility with different sterilization processes and affect sterilization efficacy Design issues (e.g. screws, hinges) will also affect sterilization efficacy

What are the monitors for validating the sterilization procedure?

The sterilization procedure should be monitored routinely by:
- Mechanical indicators: Time, temperature and pressure
- Chemical indicators: Class 1 to Class 6
- Biological indicators.

Explanation[1]

Mechanical Indicator

Mechanical monitors for steam sterilization include the daily assessment of cycle either by manual recording or computer printout and the records need to be maintained:
- Time
- Temperature
- Pressure.

Chemical Indicators

Chemical indicators are convenient, inexpensive, and indicate that the item has been exposed to the sterilization process.

Chemical indicators have been grouped into six classes based on their ability to monitor one or multiple sterilization parameters:

- **Class 1:** They are process indicators, which show that the unit has been exposed directly to steam, e.g., indicator tapes, indicator labels that should be put outside every pack
- **Class 2:** This is Bowie Dick test used for equipment control to evaluate the efficacy of air removal and steam sterilization in dynamic air removal sterilizers
- **Class 3:** A single variable indicator is of not much use
- **Class 4:** Multivariable indicators are used for pack control monitoring and should be used inside each pack
- **Class 5:** They are integrating indicators to react to all critical variables used for pack control monitoring and placed inside each pack; they can be used to release loads, which do not contain implants
- **Class 6:** They are emulating indicators.

The class 1, 2 and 5 are important indicators that help in monitoring.

Chemical indicators usually are either heat- or chemical-sensitive inks that change color, when one or more sterilization parameters (e.g. steam sterilization—time, temperature and/or saturated steam; ETO sterilization—time, temperature, relative humidity and/or ETO concentration) are present.

Biological Indicators

Biological indicators are the only process indicators that directly monitor the lethality of a given sterilization process.

An ideal biological monitor of the sterilization process should be easy to use, inexpensive, not be subject to exogenous contamination, provide positive results as soon as possible after the cycle, so that corrective action may be accomplished and provide positive results only when the sterilization parameters (as mentioned above) are inadequate to kill microbial contaminates.

Biological indicators are to be used on daily basis or at least weekly basis and when implants are loaded.

Bacillus atrophaeus spores (10^6) are used to monitor ETO and dry heat sterilization and are incubated at 35–37°C.

Geobacillus stearothermophilus spores (10^5) are used to monitor steam sterilization, hydrogen peroxide gas plasma and liquid peracetic acid sterilizers, and are incubated at 55–60°C.

Steam and low temperature sterilizers (e.g. hydrogen peroxide gas plasma, peracetic acid) should be monitored at least weekly with the appropriate commercial preparation of spores. Each load should be monitored if it contains implantable objects.

What is the optimum method of sterilization of lumen (e.g. arthroscopy) instruments, which cannot be autoclaved?

The optimum method for arthroscopy instruments is sterilization with the following:
- **Ethylene oxide sterilization:**
  - **Advantages:** It is highly diffusive and excellent penetration. Items can be packed in plastic pouches, giving a long shelf life.
  - **Disadvantages:** It is a highly inflammable and explosive gas. Lengthy procedure (12–16 hours) and requires aeration to remove adsorbed gas from sterile articles.
- **Plasma sterilizer:**
  - **Advantages:** About 95% of the medical devices are compatible with hydrogen peroxide (H_2O_2) plasma, time taken is less (60–70 minutes), no aeration required.
- They can also be disinfected with high level disinfection, e.g., Cidex (glutaraldehyde).

Formalin chambers are not to be used. Steam autoclave is also to be avoided, as extremes of temparature may cause loosening of lenses.

Explanation[1]

As with laparoscopes and other equipment that enter sterile body sites, arthroscopes ideally should be sterilized before used.

There still exists controversy with respect to use of high level disinfection versus sterilization for arthroscopes/laryngoscopes. Proponents of high level disinfection claim that only few organisms are introduced in the body by these instruments, the soft tissue damage is much less, the natural bioburden is quite less on these lumened instruments, incidence of infection is quite low in such cases and disinfection is enough to tackle common organisms. Proponents of sterilization claim risk of transmitting spores and sterlization as standard procedure for all instruments that enter sterile body cavities. This debate will continue till more robust evidence is available, however high level disinfectant can be considered as current standard.

How are the sterile instruments transported from CSSD to operation theater (OT) ward/casualty?

Sterility is event related and is dependent on the amount of handling, the conditions during transportation and storage, and the quality of the packaging material.[4]

Sterile items should be transported in covered or enclosed trolleys with solid-bottom shelves and brakes should be present. The trolley should be cleaned and disinfected after each use.

SUMMARY

1. Disinfection and sterilization are essential for ensuring that medical and surgical instruments do not transmit infectious pathogens to patients.

2. Steam sterilizer (pre vacuum type) is the most common method used for sterilization of instruments and linen.
3. Ethylene oxide sterilization and H_2O_2 gas plasma sterilization has been the most commonly used process for sterilizing temperature and moisture-sensitive medical devices.
4. CSSD should not have a dirty/washing area, packing area and sterile store room for storing sterile instruments after sterilization.
5. The sterilization procedure should be monitored routinely by mechanical indicators, chemical indicators and biological indicators.

REFERENCES

1. Rutala WA, Weber DJ. Healthcare Infection Control Practices Advisory Committee (HICPAC). (2008). CDC-Guidelines for disinfection and sterilization in healthcare facilities. [online]. Available from http://www.cdc.gov/hicpac/Disinfection_sterilization/toc.html [Accessed] September, 2014.
2. Training Manual for Health Care Central Service Technicians, 5th Edition. American Society for Healthcare Central Services Professionals; November 2005.
3. Association for Advancement of Medical Instrumentation. ANSI/AAMI ST79:2010 and A1 and A2; 2011. p. 67.
4. Recommended practices for sterilization. Perioperative Standards and Recommended Practices. Denver, CO: AORN, Inc: 2013. pp. 513-40.

2
Operation Theater Planning and Protocols

Sancheti KH, Ali J Electricwala, Bharat S Mody, Rajasekaran S

INTRODUCTION

Surgical site infection (SSI) is the second most common healthcare-associated infection. Surgical site infection accounts for 14–16% of hospital-acquired infections. Reported SSI rates ranged from 0.5 to 13%, depending on the type of surgery and patient characteristics.

Although designing of the operation theater (OT) complex has been influenced by the needs of modern surgical and anesthetic equipments and techniques, the planning of operation theaters has been dominated more by tradition. Improvement in surgical equipments and an increased appreciation of the methods by which infections spread, makes it timely that the conventional methods of OT planning meet the present day requirements so that modifications in accepted planning methods could contribute to asepsis and ease of working.

Applying strategies for the prevention of surgical site infection help to reduce surgical patients' morbidity, mortality and length of stay, and saves cost for the healthcare institutions.

Objectives of OT planning are as follows:
- To promote the highest standards of asepsis
- To ensure maximum safety for patients and staff from installation hazards
- Optimum utilization of OT and staff time

- Smooth and effective functioning of the OT
- Good working environment for the doctors and staff.

Planning of work zones in OT complex is of utmost importance from the standpoint of infection control and maintenance of ideal OT working environment. The work zones within the OT complex must be planned under the following heads:

- Central sterile supply department (CSSD) and OT store
- Changing area and washroom, doctor's lounge
- Sterile corridors and unsterile corridors
- Preoperative hold and induction room
- Operating theaters
- Recovery.

Built up space required for a modern day orthopedic OT complex:

- Operating theater—400 square feet
- CSSD—800 square feet
- Doctor's room, change area and washroom—200 square feet
- Induction room—200 square feet
- Associated corridors—350 square feet
- Doctor's lounge and OT store—150–300 square feet
- Recovery—300 square feet.

Therefore, 2,500 square feet is the base minimum carpet area required for one OT complex in Indian scenario.

Is zoning of the CSSD recommended?

It is recommended that the CSSD be zoned into sterile, clean and soiled areas separated by barriers. The administrative and storage area must be located in the clean zone; the autoclaving area, sterile storage and issue areas must be located in the sterile zone.

Explanation[1-3]

Zoning within the CSSD enables separate entries for sterile, clean and soiled materials and equipments. There should be a strict separation of staff working in the three different areas. There must be a positive pressure air gradient of minimum 15 Pascal between the CSSD and the adjoining areas.

Points to Note

For the Indian scenario, it may not be feasible to have a positive pressure air handling in the entire CSSD. Hence, it would suffice to have a positive pressure air handling only in the sterile zone of the CSSD. Moreover the sterile storage area of the CSSD may be a part of the sterile zone of the main OT complex. This would eliminate the need to have a separate air-handling unit (AHU) for the CSSD and thereby minimize the cost.

Zoning of the OT Complex

In order to provide maximum asepsis the entire OT complex can be divided into various zones:
- **Protective zone**
- **Clean zone**
- **Aseptic zone**
- **Disposal zone.**

Protective zone includes:
- Reception, patient identification and case sheet check
- Waiting area for relatives
- Changing room for the OT staff and surgeons
- Pre-anesthesia checkup room
- Store room, trolley room
- Record and controller room
- OT in charge desk
- Seminar and meeting room
- Entrance to observation gallery.

Clean zone includes:
- Patient preparation room
- Recovery room

- Plaster room, blood storage and frozen section
- Doctor's lounge
- Induction room
- Equipment room, drugs, intravenous (IV) lines
- Administrative area of CSSD
- Storage area of CSSD.

Sterile or aseptic zone includes:
- Operating room (OR)
- Sterile corridor
- Scrub station
- Anesthesia station
- Instrument station
- Autoclave, sterile storage and issue area of CSSD.

Disposal zone includes:
- Washroom
- Unsterile corridor.

What is the recommended floor and wall coating of the CSSD?

It is recommended that the CSSD floors can be made from any one of the following materials:
- Epoxy coating
- Kota stone.

It is recommended that the CSSD walls be coated with polyurethane or ceramic/vitrified glazed tiles.

Explanation[4-8]

Epoxy coated flooring provides a horizontal smooth surface, strong enough to bear heavy loads and easy to clean. Polyurethane coated walls are resistant to dust settling and are easy to clean.

Epoxy is the cured end product of epoxy resins, as well as a colloquial name for the epoxide functional group. Epoxy is also a common name for a type of strong adhesive used for sticking things together and covering surfaces typically two resins that need to be mixed together before use. Epoxy resins, also known as polyepoxides are a class of reactive prepolymers and polymers, which contain epoxide groups. Epoxy resins are cross-linked to make them smooth, hard and strong.

Points to Note

Whilst epoxy is suitable for an area like the CSSD, where dropping of instruments and various liquid chemicals can cause breakage and damage to the floor, and epoxy is resistant to this event; kota stone is another less expensive and equally appropriate flooring material because of the following qualities:

- It is dense, hard and nonporous
- It can be polished to a high level of finish
- It can be laid with seamless joinery
- It is relatively inexpensive (₹ 60 per square feet inclusive of most cost headings), the expertise is available widely in all parts of the country.

Polyurethane-based coatings are characterized by a specifically adaptable 'hard-soft-segmentation,' which results in good flexibility over a large range of temperatures. Consequently, small cracks can be bridged better compared to coating systems based on other raw materials. Moreover, polyurethane coatings show a good solvent and chemical resistance, which provides durable protection for a long time. Other materials that can be used are ceramic/vitrified glazed tiles. This material allows aggressive cleaning with acidic/alkaline solutions. It is stain resistant. It is inexpensive and widely available (₹ 40 per square feet) whilst it does have the creation of unsterile joints, this feature is not critically important in CSSD.

Should there be a separate sterile and unsterile corridor?

It is recommended that there should be a separate sterile corridor connecting the preoperative hold to the operating rooms and an unsterile corridor connecting the operating rooms to the disposal zone whenever possible.

> **Explanation**

The centralized sterile unit should be as close to the OT as possible, its position being influence be the need to have access from the hospital to the stores adjoining the preparation room and from the disposal bay to the hospital circulation. These communications should be horizontal or vertical. To obtain a smoothly flowing circulation of sterile goods from the sterilizing rooms to the theater supply rooms and of soiled articles to the disposal zone, it is expedient to provide separate sterile and unsterile corridors. One route should be along the theater corridor and the other could be by a separate passage reserved for movement of trolleys in one direction only. This passage should be used for sterile goods to avoid risk of contamination and to shorten the journey to the theater. Soiled articles would be returned to the disposal room using a separate unsterile corridor. They should be covered with polythene drapes to prevent air-borne spread of infection during the transit and to conceal anything, which might distress the patient on the way to the postoperative recovery room. A sink must be present near the exit from each theater for cleaning the operation floor and table in between cases.

The unsterile trolley must be transported in a unidirectional way using the unsterile corridor to the disposal bay.

Points to Note

It may not be always feasible to have separate sterile and unsterile corridors, as it requires all the operating rooms in one line.

Whilst separate sterile and unsterile corridors would be the ideal setup, in reality it would often be the case wherein the size of the land and the orientation of the building plans might not allow this feature to be included in the space planning. Given this condition, it would suffice to ensure minimum crossing of postprocedure disposal of dirty material through sterile areas. Further, sealed plastic binning of the dirty material before evacuating them from the OT will prevent the violation of sterility of the sterile areas during their movements.

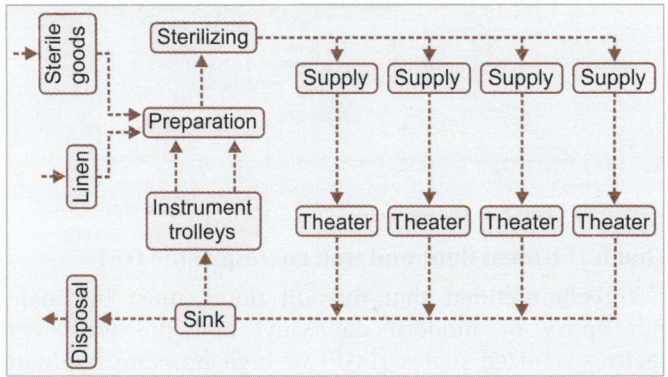

Fig. 2.1: Plan showing sterilizing and sink rooms removed from the vicinity of the operation theater[11]

What is the recommended size of the OR?

It is recommended that the standard size of the OR is 20 × 20 square feet with 10 feet height from below the level of false ceiling.

Explanation[4,7-10]

The standard size of the operating table is 6 × 2 feet. Approximately 7 feet of working space is needed on all sides of the operating table. The anesthesia machine requires a minimum of 10 square feet at the head end of the table. An additional 4 feet of space, which remains on two sides of the operating table is used to accommodate materials that are necessary for surgery, e.g., prosthesis, suture material, IV bottles, etc.

The bare minimum top of concrete (TOC) to TOC distance required is approximately 4.2 meters to accommodate OT lamps, AHU, etc.

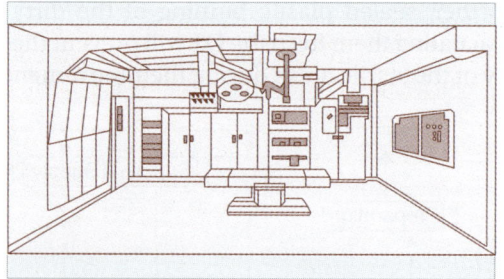

Fig. 2.2: Different areas in operation theater (OT)

What is the ideal floor and wall coating of the OR?

It is recommended that the OR floors must be coated with epoxy or modern day vinyl and the walls with electrogalvanized plates (EGP) or high pressure laminates (HPL) or polyurethane.

Explanation

Epoxy Coating of Floors

Epoxy coating of floors provides a horizontal smooth surface, which is strong enough to bear heavy loads and easy to clean. Polyurethane coated walls are resistant to dust settling, less light reflecting, washable and easy to clean.

Epoxy is the cured end product of epoxy resins, as well as a colloquial name for the epoxide functional group. Epoxy is also a common name for a type of strong adhesive used for sticking things together and covering surfaces typically two resins that need to be mixed together before use. Epoxy resins, also known as polyepoxides are a class of reactive prepolymers and polymers, which contain epoxide groups. Epoxy resins are cross-linked to make them smooth, hard and strong.

Points to Note
Epoxy has the following shortcomings:
- Epoxy comes in a fluid state and its application requires a very highly skilled labor force if the aim is to get a perfectly leveled and microundulation free surface. This is not easy to obtain in all parts of the country. Its use in the industrial flooring is not constrained by this issue.
- Epoxy as a material is usually very dull in color and is always in a monotone. This has an impact on the overall ambience in the OR.

Vinyl/Linoleum Flooring
Vinyl/Linoleum flooring category comes in tiles/rolls. It is easy to apply and there are special grades available for hospital and OR use. These have features such as stain resistance, electroconductivity, seamless joinery, vibrant color shades, 2 mm or 3 mm homogeneous thickness, etc. They can be applied very rapidly. The material and the skill sets for application are widely available now in India.

Electrogalvanized Powder Coated Sheets
Electrogalvanized powder coated sheets provide a seamless surface. The positives are relatively less expensive, vendors available in abundance. The disadvantages are: Can dent on impact and surface not as microundulation free as HPL.

High Pressure Laminates
High pressure laminates are highly polished surfaces available in the form of 2 mm sheets constructed as polyurethane foam (PUF) panels. These are typically used in the construction of clean air facilities for high end microelectronics manufacturing facility and/or critical pharmaceutical formulation facility. The advantages of HPL are—no microundulations, seamless, stain resistant, dent resistant, vibrant colors available, rapid construction possible, etc. The disadvantages are: Limited vendors and costly material.

Polyurethane based coatings are characterized by a specifically adaptable 'hard-soft-segmentation' which results in good flexibility over a large range of temperatures. Consequently, small cracks can be bridged better compared to coating systems based on other raw materials. Moreover, polyurethane coatings show a good solvent and chemical resistance, which provides durable protection for a long time.

Cowing of walls of the OR is recommended to prevent accumulation of dust particles and to allow easy cleaning.

Suitable Materials for Floor Coatings

- Epoxy
- Modern day vinyl coated over a subsurface of modern day Kota stone or self-leveling fluid
- High pressure laminates
- Electrogalvanized plates
- Stainless steel
- Polyurethane.

Doors in the OT should be sliding or hinge?

It is recommended that doors of the OR must be sliding.

Explanation

Hinge doors are air pushing and therefore generate air currents within the OR. Sliding doors are air cutting and hence are recommended.

What is the ideal temperature and humidity within the OR?

It is recommended to maintain temperature at 18–23°C and relative humidity at 30–60%.

Explanation[3,4,11-14]

It is necessary to maintain optimum OR temperature and relative humidity to minimize perspiration, bacterial colonization and also for the comfort of the surgeon, anesthetist and patient. Therefore an OR temperature of 18–23°C and relative humidity of 30–60% is recommended.

What is the ideal pressure gradient within the OR?

It is recommended to maintain positive pressure gradient between the OR and the adjoining areas and corridors. A minimum pressure gradient of 15 Pascal (0.05 inch of water) is recommended.

Explanation

Positive pressure gradient between the OR and the adjoining areas prevents entry of outside air into the OR. However, a program of periodic checking and system maintenance is important to ensure that the target pressure gradient is maintained and that out of range performance can be detected.

A positive pressure gradient of 15 Pascal is monitored by differential pressure gauge.

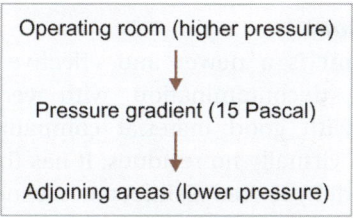

What is the recommended operating light intensity?

It is recommended that the operating light must be shadowless, mobile, hanging from the ceiling and easily maintainable. The intensity should be 4,000 lux at the incision site and 8,000 lux at 9 cm deep.

What should be the sterilization protocol of the modern day OR?

It is recommended that the OR must be sterilized once a week (end of the week sterilization) with hydrogen peroxide and Bacillocid. In case of an infected case, it is recommended that the OR is sterilized at the end of the case.[14]

Samples from the OR must be sent once in a week for culture and from minimum of five sites within the OR premises (operating table, OT lamp, suction machine, tourniquet, Boyle's apparatus, and image intensifier).

Formaldehyde is a potential carcinogen and is no longer recommended for OR sterilization.

Other agents such as hydrogen peroxide, hydrogen peroxide with silver nitrate, peracetic acid and other chemical compounds of formaldehyde should be used in place of currently prevalent practice of using formaldehyde. These agents are dispersed with the help of a fogger-like device inside the OR environment. The recommended contact time is 1 hour and the OR may be used immediately after the contact time.

Bacillocid Rasant

Bacillocid rasant is a newer and effective compound in environmental decontamination with very good cost-benefit ratio with good material compatibility, cleaning properties and virtually no residues. It has the advantage of being a formaldehyde-free disinfectant cleaner with low use concentration.

Active ingredients are—gluteal, benzyl-C12-18-alkyldimethyl ammonium chloride.

Advantages
- Provides complete asepsis within 30–60 minutes
- Cleaning with detergent or carbolic acid is not required
- Formaldehyde fumigation is not required
- Shutdown of OR for 24 hours is not required.

SUMMARY

1. Proper planning of work zones within the OT complex and maintenance of OR decorum is of utmost importance from the standpoint of infection control.

2. Exert traffic control of OR by restricting the number of people allowed in the OR, closing the doors to the OR to prevent in and out traffic, and limiting unnecessary movement and silence should be maintained in the OR.
3. Maintain positive-pressure ventilation for operating rooms with respect to corridors and adjacent areas. A program for periodic checking and system maintenance assessment is important to ensure that the target pressure gradient is maintained and that out of range performance can be detected.
4. Maintain relative humidity at 30–60% and temperature at 18–23°C.
5. Separate sterile and unsterile corridors within the OT complex are recommended.
6. Standard size of the OR is 20 × 20 square feet with 10 feet height from below the level of false ceiling.
7. Epoxy coating of the walls and polyurethane coating of the floors of the OR and CSSD is recommended.
8. It is recommended that the operating light must be shadowless, mobile, hanging from the ceiling and easily maintainable. The intensity should be 4,000 lux at the incision site and 8,000 lux at 9 cm deep.
9. Formaldehyde is a potential carcinogen and is no longer recommended for OR sterilization.

REFERENCES

1. Dorsch JA, Dorsch SE. Operating room design and equipment selection. In: Dorsch JA, Dorsch SE (Eds). Understanding Anesthesia Equipment, 4th edition. Williams and Wilkins; 1999. pp. 1015-6.
2. Barash PG, Cullen BF, Stoelting RK. Value based anesthesia practice, resource utilisation and operating room management. In: Barash PG, Cullen BF, Stoelting RK (Eds).Clinical Anaesthesia, 4th edition. Lippincott: Williams and Wilkins; 2001. pp. 111-2.
3. Gupta SK, Kant S, Chandrashekhar R. Operating unit—planning essentials and design considerations. Journal of Academy of Hospital Administration. 2005;17:01-12.
4. Bridgen RJ. Ch.1. The Operating department 2. Organisation and Management 3. Electricity and Electromedical Equipment

4. Static Electricity: Operating theater technique, 5th edition. Churchill Livingstone 1988; 09, 10, 13, 16-21, 27-31, 41, 43-45, 109.
5. Moyle JTB, Davey A, Ward CS. The anaesthetic room and recovery area. In: Miller RD (Ed). Ward's Anaesthetic Equipment, 3rd edition. WB Saunder's; 1992. pp. 347-51.
6. Miller RD. Operating room information systems. In: Miller RD (Ed). Miller's Anesthesia, 6th edition. Churchill Livingstone: Elsevier; 2005. pp. 3131-2.
7. Joint Commission on Accreditation of Healthcare Organizations. [online]. Available from www.jointcommission.org/AccreditationPrograms/Hospitals/
8. Bartley JM. APIC state-of-the-Art report: the role of infection control during construction in health care facilities. Am J Infect Control. 2000;28(2):156-69.
9. Shine TSJ, Leone BJ, Martin DL. Specialized Operating Rooms. Operating Room Design Manual: American Society of Anesthesiologist; 2012. pp. 44-56.
10. Bartley J, Olmsted RN. Construction and renovation. In: Carrico R (Ed). APIC Text of Infection control and Epidemiology, 3rd edition. Washington, DC: Association for Professionals in Infection Control and Epidemiology, Inc; 2009. p. 106.
11. Michael Essex-Lopresti, David Hubert. Planning operating-theatre suites. Br Med J. 1962;1(5290):1470-3.
12. Streifel AJ. Design and maintenance of hospital ventilation systems and the prevention of airborne nosocomial infections. In: Mayhall CG (Ed). Hospital Epidemiology and Infection Control. Baltimore: Williams and Wilkins; 2004. pp. 1577-89.
13. Heating and ventilation of health sector buildings (HTM 03-01). [online]. Available from www.gov.uk/government/publications/guidance-on-specialised-ventilation-for-healthcare-premises-parts-a-and-b [Accessed November, 2007].
14. American Society of Healthcare Engineering of the American Hospital Association, Chicago. (2010). Facility Guidelines Institute. Guidelines for design and construction of health care facilities. [online]. Available from www.fgiguidelines.org

3
Surgeon Preparation and Scrubbing Protocols

Vivek Vincent Valiyaveettil, Gurava Reddy, Ashok Shyam, Parag K Sancheti

INTRODUCTION

Surgical site infections (SSIs) greatly contribute to nosocomial infections. Some of the risk factors for nosocomial infections include the behavior of personnel regarding decontamination practices, hand hygiene/antisepsis and compliance with universal precautions. Most surgical professionals agree on the importance of good surgical handwashing practices in infection prevention. Hand bacterial transmission is a critical factor in the spreading of bacteria, pathogens and viruses that cause disease and nosocomial infections in general. Here are few recommendations regarding surgeon preparations.

What are the present recommendation standards for surgeon attire in OT?

- **Head and face:** Operation theater (OT) caps and face masks
- **Eyes:** Eyewear, which completely covers the eyes should be used to avoid any blood spillage into the eyes
- **Hands:** Double gloves for each surgery
- **Body:** OT gowns covering the entire body; the gowns can be disposable or nondisposable
- **Footwear:** Rubber boots with impervious soles are must.

Explanation

Gowns and drapes should be resistant to liquid penetration and also, resistant to microbial penetration with a minimal release of particles. Disposable, polypropylene spun bound laminate materials should be used. Well-fitting footwear with impervious soles should be worn and regularly cleaned to remove splashes of blood and body fluid.[1,2] All footwear should be cleaned after every use. Rubber boots are recommended. Protective gear, in the form of glasses and hoods, should be used for each case. Wearing of double gloves at surgical procedures protects the surgeon from viral transmission. Two pairs of gloves decreases leaks by 3–9 fold in water permeability tests. Gloves acts as a barrier for personal protection from patient's blood and exudates and prevents bacteria from surgeon's hands entering the surgical site. Use of masks with a filter size of less than 1.1 μm should be worn over mouth and nose with visor or goggles for protection. Fresh mask should be worn for each operation and masks that become damp should be replaced. Well-fitting footwear with impervious soles should be worn and regularly cleaned to remove splashes of blood and body fluid. All footwear should be cleaned after every use. Hoods and glasses should be used to protect the eyes from any blood spillage or any form of injury during and operative procedure.

Are disposable gowns mandatory?

No, disposable gowns are not mandatory for all orthopedic surgical cases. Spunbonded meltdown spunbonded (SMS) gowns are considered a good option for disposable gowns in terms of water repellent and durability. We recommend usage of non-disposable gowns in term of cost management and waste management however, quality of the gown should be maintained.

Explanation

Gowns and drapes should be resistant to liquid penetration, resistant to microbial penetration with a minimal release of particles. Disposable, polypropylene spunbond laminate materials should be used. Disposable gowns reduce the amount of surgical waste, are environment friendly and also cost effective. Well-fitting footwear with impervious soles should be worn and regularly cleaned to remove splashes of blood and body fluid.[3] All footwear should be cleaned after every use. Rubber boots are recommended. Protective gear, in the form of glasses and hoods, should be used for each case. Wearing two pairs of gloves (double gloving) has been shown to reduce hand contact with patient's blood and body fluids when compared to wearing only a single pair and also decreases chances of nosocomial infections.[4]

What are the prerequisites for an OT gown?

Clothing made from hydrophobic, spunlaced 70 g/m^2, polyester pulp non-woven material with mesh size less than 80 microns is effective and more comfortable and convenient to wear.[4-6]

What is the optimal duration of handwash time and ideal antiseptic required before operation?

An initial 2 or 3 minute scrub with 4% chlorhexidine gluconate or 7.5% povidone-iodine (either solution is good) followed by application of an alcohol-based product (example sterillium etc.) has been as effective as a 5-minute scrub with an antiseptic detergent.[7,8,9] After this, hands have to be dried with a sterile towel or napkin. Alcoholic scrub must be used after handwash. The alcoholic hand rub should be completely dried off before wearing gloves. It is recommended to use potable water for handwashing while scrubbing. Chlorhexidine and povidone-iodine have been considered ideal antiseptic agents, which can be used for scrubbing. Alcoholic hand rubs are highly effective in killing microorganisms on skin surfaces. Ethanol or isopropanol 60–80% is more effective than detergents or antiseptic soaps.

> **Explanation**

An ideal antiseptic should be a broad spectrum antiseptic against gram-negative and gram-positive bacteria resistant from organic materials such as feces and blood. The most effective agent for reducing bacterial count immediately after hand disinfection are formulations containing 60–95% alcohol alone or 50–95% when combined with chlorhexidine gluconate. These are followed by, in order of decreasing activity, chlorhexidine gluconate, iodophors, triclosan and plain soap.[9] Originally an handwash duration of 10 minutes was advised for surgeons in orthopedic surgeries, however, studies have noted that these may cause skin damage and may actually increase bacterial shedding.[7,8] A 5-minute handwash is found to be effective with minimum three times application rinse cycle. It is recommended that brush or sponge are not to be used also hot water is not to be used for handwash (warm water interferes microbial activities of the antiseptics).[9]

Are there any differences in preparation for a human immunodeficiency virus (HIV) patient in comparison to other surgical patients?

There is are no differences in preparing a routine patient from an HIV patient. Each patient should be treated and draped as if an HIV patient. However, if the HIV test is done and is positive then universal precautions should be undertaken (eyewear, double gloves and gum boots).

> **Explanation**

Double gloving, protective eyewear and boots actually should be used for each case as an HIV patients can be in their window period. To avoid any complications the surgeon must have complete surgical attire on for each and every case of surgery.

SUMMARY

1. Protective gear in form of cap, mask, eye wear, double gloves, gowns and boots with impervious soles are essential gear for all surgeries.
2. Gowns and drapes should be resistant to liquid penetration, resistant to microbial penetration with a minimal release of particles. They need not always be disposable, but standard requirements in terms of fabric and pore size should be followed.
3. Handwash should be a three step process with 1 minute of 4% chlorhexidine gluconate followed by 2–3 minutes of 7.5% povidine-iodine, which is dried. Alcohol based rub is used and dried completely before wearing the gloves. A two step use of povidine iodine for 3 minutes (two washes) and subsequent use of alcohol based rub is also sufficient for routine orthopedic cases.
4. Potable water should be used for handwash preferably; hot water should not be used.

REFERENCES

1. Woodhead K, Taylor EW, Bannister G, et al. Behaviours and rituals in the operating theatre. A report from the Hospital Infection Society Working Party on Infection Control in Operating Theaters. H Hosp Infect. 2002;51(4):241-55.
2. Doyle PM, Alvi S, Johanson R. The effectiveness of double-gloving in obstetrics and gynaecology. Br J Obstet Gynaecol. 1992;99(1):83-4.
3. Dodds RD, Guy PJ, Peacock AM, et al. Surgical glove perforation. Br J Surg. 1988;75(10):966-8.
4. Mitchell NJ, Evans DS, Kerr A. Reduction of skin bacteria in theatre air with comfortable, non-woven disposable clothing for operating-theatre staff. Br Med J. 1978;1(6114):696-8.
5. Tammelin A, Ljungqvist B, Reinmüller B. Single-use surgical clothing system for reduction of airborne bacteria in the operating room. J Hosp Infect. 2013;84(3):245-7.
6. Blom AW, Barnett A, Ajitsaria P, Noel A, Estela CM. Resistance of disposable drapes to bacterial penetration. J OrthopSurg (Hong Kong). 2007 Dec;15(3):267-9.

7. Boyce JM, Pittet D. Healthcare Infection Control Practices Advisory Committee;HICPAC/SHEA/APIC/IDSA Hand Hygiene Task Force. Guideline for Hand Hygiene in Health-Care Settings. Recommendations of the Healthcare Infection Control Practices Advisory Committee and the HICPAC/SHEA/APIC/IDSA Hand Hygiene Task Force. Am J Infect Control. 2002;30(8):S1-46.
8. World Health Organization. (2009). WHO Guidelines on Hand Hygiene in Health Care. [online]. Available from http://whqlibdoc.who.int/publications/2009/978924/1597906_eng.pdf
9. Nicolay CR. Hand hygiene: an evidence-based review for surgeons. Int J Surg. 2006;4(1):53-65.

4
Laminar Airflow and Air-handling Unit

Sancheti KH, Ali J Electricwala, Rajasekaran S, Bharat S Mody

INTRODUCTION

Proper ventilation and maintenance of operating room (OR) environment is necessary for prevention of surgical site infections (SSIs).

SSIs, a leading complication of surgery, is particularly devastating and expensive to treat when it occurs in orthopedic implant surgery. With the current trend toward pay-for-performance standards, orthopedic surgeons must consider taking advantage of all available potential infection control measures. Both airborne bacteria and other sources of bacterial contamination must be reduced to a minimum to achieve optimal SSI rates.

Several studies have shown a reduced infection rate in orthopedic implant surgeries performed in ultraclean air facilities and body exhaust suits. Over the decades of laminar flow OR, ventilation in combination with other infection, control measures have improved infection rates; however, no uniform opinion about laminar flow efficacy has developed.[1-7]

Laminar airflow results in a statistically significant reduction in airborne bacterial colony forming units (CFU); a decrease in infection rates with statistical significance has not been shown. This is due to the number of uncontrolled variables in OR infection control. The Centers for Disease Control and Prevention (CDC) also confirms that variables during multiple evaluations of laminar flow may have 'confounded the associations'. Based on this, some surgeons have disputed the results of studies showing laminar flow efficacy.

Uncontrolled variables include improved air turnover in traditional ORs, standardization of prophylactic antibiotics, behavioral change in personnel and awareness, and elimination of other vectors of wound contamination.

LAMINAR AIRFLOW IN THE OPERATING ROOM

Laminar flow (or streamline flow) occurs when a fluid flows in parallel layer with no cross-currents, eddies or disruptions. Laminar airflow is intended to provide uniform, directional airflow that essentially 'moves' particles floating in the airstream away from areas that are intended to be contaminant-free (i.e. the sterile field) to where they can be disposed of and contained (through the return ducts and filtration system). Turbulence is undesirable because particles are allowed to float undirected, eliminating any ability to predict where they may settle.

Laminar flow technology itself has evolved through the years. Improvement of laminar flow technology has presented its own evaluation challenge. This technology has evolved from fiberglass wall packs to high-efficiency particulate air (HEPA) filtration systems. HEPA-filtered laminar airflow can be provided by vertical airflow systems and by unidirectional horizontal flow from wall-mounted units, with and without curtains or sliding walls. Because each system has its own associated problems of airflow disruption, newer 'exponential laminar flow' systems have been developed in which the airflow takes the form of an upside-down trumpet. It is difficult to establish specific system comparisons and recommendations, however, because studies that document the merits of any one system do not include system design data. For airflow to be laminar the velocity of air must be 9 meter per second.

High Efficiency Particulate Air Filters

The 'HEPA' is an acronym, which stands for high efficiency particulate air. HEPA filters provide a very high level of filtration efficiency for the smallest as well as the largest particulate contaminants. As defined by the Institute of Environmental Sciences and Technology, a HEPA filter must capture a minimum of 99.7% of contaminants at 0.3 microns in size. The 0.3 micron benchmark is used in efficiency ratings, because it approximates the most difficult particle size for a filter to capture. HEPA filters are even more efficient in removing particles that are smaller than 0.3 microns and larger than 0.3 microns. The fact that a HEPA filter's removal efficiency increases as particle size below 0.3 microns is counter intuitive. However, this is a proven and accepted fact in the filtration sciences. The filtration mechanisms below explains how a HEPA filter does this.

Function of a HEPA Filter

A HEPA filter is used in an air purifier to help filter harmful pollutants and allergens out of the air you breathe. This technology was developed by the United States Atomic Energy Commission to remove the airborne radioactive particles from the air. In order for a filter to be considered a true HEPA, it has to be able to remove 99.7% of the particles as small as 0.3 microns from the air.

There are several different categories of HEPA filters:
- **True HEPA filters:** These filters are tested to ensure they will filter with 99.7% efficiency. They must have seal attached to them certifying that they have been tested with a serial number and the test results are printed here as well. They are more expensive and must perform to the standard.

- **HEPA type filters:** They look much like the true filters, but are not tested to perform to the 99.7% efficiency rate. They are not as expensive and will only capture 85–90% of the particles in the air.

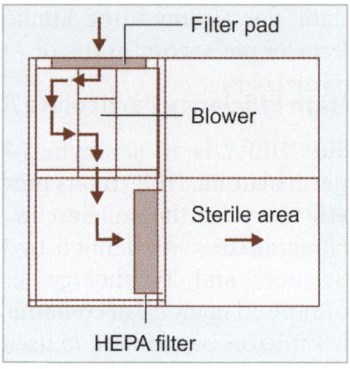

Fig. 4.1: Laminar airflow system and high efficiency particulate air (HEPA) filters used in operation theater

High efficiency particulate air filters trap small particles in the air. The more square feet you have in the filter media, the more particles it can remove from the air before it needs to be changed. It will also be able to remove more impurities from the air each time it passes over filter. It is very important to have a good quality filter because the pleats need to be uniform to give each one the same filtration efficiency. If the pleats are too close together they may actually restrict the airflow and there will not be as much airflow as you need.

The material used in the filter is very important. Some filters use synthetic material, but thin paper is the best. It is the most effective at removing the harmful particles without restricting the airflow. This material is easy to damage when operator handling it, so the air purifier has to be designed in such a way that it also protects the filter.

Most air filters use a method called impingement to purify the air and trap the airborne particles. HEPA air filters use this method by using fine materials such as thin paper through which they draw the air. The particles in the air become trapped on the material and the air that flows back into the room is clean.

There are drawbacks on relying totally on a HEPA filter to purify the air in home or office. They cannot capture any particles that are smaller than 0.3 microns and do not treat things such as gases, odors and viruses. Because the air must pass through a filter, it is hard to purify the air in a large room. Because they need to be constantly exchanging the air, they also tend to be noisy. Even though many different types of air purifiers have been developed, most experts tend to rely on the HEPA filter as being the most effective.[8]

Recommendations regarding OR traffic control, positive pressure ventilation and laminar airflow systems, use of HEPA filters and ideal OR temperature, humidity and OR air pressure gradient have been given below to achieve the above mentioned objective.[9,10]

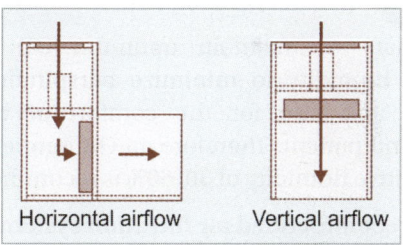

Fig. 4.2: Types of laminar airflow hoods

Is positive pressure ventilation for ORs necessary?

It is recommended to maintain positive pressure gradient between the OR and the adjoining areas, and corridors. A minimum pressure gradient of 15 Pascal (0.05 inch of water) is recommended.

Explanation

Positive pressure gradient between the OR and the adjoining areas prevents entry of outside air into the OR. However, a program of periodic checking and system maintenance is important to ensure that the target pressure gradient is maintained and that out of range performance can be detected.[11-14]

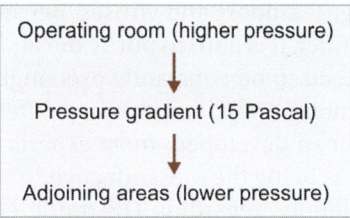

What is the ideal temperature and humidity of the OR?

It is recommended to maintain temperature at 18°C–23°C and relative humidity at 30–60%.

Explanation

It is necessary to maintain optimum OR temperature and relative humidity to minimize perspiration, bacterial colonization and also for the comfort of the surgeon, anesthetist and patient. Therefore an OR temperature of 18–23°C and relative humidity of 30–60% is recommended.[13-15]

What is the recommended air filtration system?

It is recommended that all fresh air and recirculated air be filtered through HEPA filters. However, laminar airflow is not a must for orthopedic ORs.

Explanation

High efficiency particulate air filters remove at least 99.97% of airborne particles 0.3 micrometers (μm) in diameter. HEPA filters are critical in the prevention of the spread of airborne bacterial and viral organisms, and therefore, infection. Typically, medical-use HEPA filtration systems also incorporate high-energy ultraviolet light units to kill off the live bacteria and viruses trapped by the filter media. Some of the best-rated HEPA units have an efficiency rating of 99.95%, which assures a very high level of protection against airborne disease transmission.[14,16] One must understand that HEPA filters are different from laminar airflow and is recommended to be installed in all ORs.

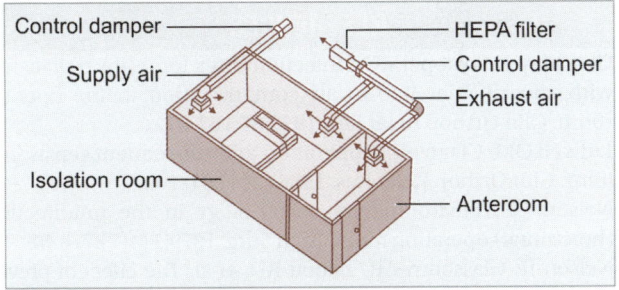

Fig. 4.3: Air filtration system

What is the recommended air handling in the OR?

Air must be introduced from the ceiling and exhaust near the floor.

Explanation

Air is supplied through HEPA filters in the air-handling unit (AHU). The minimum size of the air supply area should be 6 × 4 feet to cover the entire OT table and surgical team. The minimum supply air volume to the OT should be compliant with the desired minimum air change. The return air should be picked up/taken out from the exhaust grille located near the floor level (approximate 6 inch above the floor level).[12,13,17]

SUMMARY

1. Operating room traffic must be kept to the minimum
2. It is recommended to maintain positive pressure gradient between the OR and the adjoining areas, and corridors; a minimum pressure gradient of 15 Pascal (0.05 inch of water) is recommended

3. It is recommended to maintain temperature at 18–23°C and relative humidity at 30–60%.
4. It is recommended that all fresh air and re-circulated air be filtered through HEPA filters.
5. Air must be introduced form the ceiling and exhaust near the floor.

REFERENCES

1. Charnley J. Postoperative infection after total hip replacement with special reference to air contamination in the operating room. Clin Orthop Relat Res. 1972;87:167-87.
2. Lidwell OM. Clean air at operation and subsequent sepsis in the joint. Clin Orthop Relat Res. 1986;(211):91-102.
3. Nelson CL. Environmental bacteriology in the unidirectional (horizontal) operating room. Arch Surg. 1979;114(7):778-82.
4. Nelson JP, Glassburn AR, Talbott RD, et al. The effect of previous surgery, operating room environment, and preventive antibiotics on postoperative infection following total hip arthroplasty. Clin Orthop Relat Res. 1980;(147):167-9.
5. Salvati EA, Robinson RP, Zino SM, et al. Infection rates after 3175 total hip and total knee replacements performed with and without a horizontal unidirectional filtered air-flow system. J Bone Joint Surg Am. 1982;64(4):525-35.
6. Franco JA, Baer H, Enneking WF. Airborne contamination in orthopedic surgery. Evaluation laminar air flow system and aspiration suit. Clin Orthop Relat Res. 1977;(122):231-43.
7. Laufman H. Air-flow effects in surgery. Arch Surg. 1979;114(7):826-30.
8. Humphreys H, Taylor EW. Operating theatre ventilation standards and the risk of postoperative infection. J Hosp Infect. 2002;50(2):85-90.
9. Chow TT, Yang XY. Ventilation performance in operating theatres against airborne infection: review of research activities and practical guidance. J Hosp Infect. 2004;56(2):85-92.
10. Lidwell OM, Elson RA, Lowbury EJ, et al. Ultraclean air and antibiotics for prevention of postoperative infection. A multicenter study of 8,052 joint replacement operations. Acta Orthop Scand. 1987;58(1):4-13.

11. Wong ES. Surgical site infection. In: Mayhall CG (Ed). Hospital Epidemiology and Infection Control, 3rd edition. Philadelphia: Lippincott Williams and Wilkins; 2004. pp. 287-310.
12. Mangram AJ, Horan TC, Pearson ML, et al. Guideline for prevention of surgical site infection. Infect Control Hosp Epidemiol. 1999;20(4):250-78.
13. Streifel AJ. Design and maintenance of hospital ventilation systems and the prevention of airborne nosocomial infections. In: Mayhall CG (Ed). Hospital Epidemiology and Infection Control, 2nd edition. Baltimore: Williams and Wilkins; 2004. pp. 1577-89.
14. Health Technical Memorandum 03-01: Specialised ventilation for healthcare premises. Part A-Design and validation and Part B-Operational management and performance verification. London: The Stationary Office; 2007.
15. American Institute of Architects. Guidelines for design and construction of hospital and health care facilities. Washington DC: American Institute of Architects Press; 2006.
16. Mechanisms of filtration for high efficiency fibrous filters. [online]. Available from http://www.tsi.com/uploaded Files/Product_Information/Literature/Application_Notes/ITI-041.pdf TSI Application Note ITI-041
17. Sehulster L, Chinn RY. Guidelines for environmental infection control in health-care facilities. MMWR Recomm Rep. 2003;52(RR-10):1-42.

5

Operation Theater Personnel

Lovey Singhal, Steve Rocha, Rajeev Joshi, Madhav Borate

INTRODUCTION

A successful surgery requires a close cooperation between many operating room personnel. They all must know their roles and responsibilities and be prepared to execute them quickly and confidently. This requires patience, empathy, time management, efficiency, and professionalism with patients and co-workers.

What are the guidelines for hand hygiene and glove use for operation theater (OT) personnel in contact with the patient for examination, manipulation and placement on the operating room (OR) table?

We recommend that OT personnel should decontaminate their hands with alcohol-based liquid solutions. If an individual is allergic to alcohol-based liquid then foam-based liquid can be used. Also, from the general consensus and available studies we suggest that gloves should be used by OT personnel as per standard precautions[1], while coming in contact with blood and body fluids.

Explanation

Hands of OT personnel can get contaminated after contact with inanimate objects in vicinity of patient.[2] All OT personnel, who deal with patient including hand hygiene application by OT staff, including anesthesiologists, anesthesia nurses, surgeons, surgical nurses and medical students should decontaminate their hands.[3] Widmer[4] suggested that hospital-acquired infections are spreaded by direct contact and it is logical to suppose that hand hygiene can interrupt the chain of infection, especially when the active ingredient in the hand hygiene agent is applied systematically to all surfaces of hands. Pettit et al[5] suggested that use of alcohol-based hand disinfectant is associated with reduced rate of nosocomial infections and methicillin-resistant *Staphylococcus aureus* (MRSA) transmission.

As per study conducted by Al-Maiyah et al[6] changing gloves after every 20 minutes and before cementing in total hip replacement surgeries led to reduction in perforation and contamination rate. Studies done by Beldame et al[7] also suggested that glove change before cementing reduces contamination rate in replacement surgeries. Kaya et al[8] suggested that gloves should be changed after every 90 minutes to reduce contamination rate. According to the study done by Laine and Aarnio,[9] in view of the critical importance of safety at work by having a sterile barrier between surgeon and patient, it is very important to use a double-gloving puncture indication system, at least in operations, where there is a high risk of glove perforation.

What strategies should be implemented to keep OT traffic to the minimum?

We recommend that OT traffic should be kept to minimum about five persons and maximum up to eight persons. Strategies like keeping the OT doors closed during surgery except as needed for passage of equipment, personnel and the patient. Limiting unnecessary movement and talking in the operating room is recommended. Training and education of the OT personnel is paramount in maintaining the OT traffic.

Explanation

Ritter et al[10] showed that bacteria count in OR air increases 3–4 folds in an OR with five people compared to empty room.

According to a study done by Panahi et al[11] traffic in the OR is a major concern during total joint arthroplasty (TJA). Implementation of strategies such as storage of instruments and components in the OR and education of OR personnel is required to reduce door openings in the OR. Andersson et al[12] suggested that traffic flow has a strong negative impact on the OR environment and it should be kept to minimum. Allo et al[13] also demonstrated the same results in their study. Lynch et al[14] showed an exponential relationship between room opening and number of personnel in the OR.

What is the kind of attire used inside OT?

We suggest that all personnel should wear clean attire including disposable mask and head cap.

Can OT dress be worn outside the OT complex?

Personnel should not wear OT attire out of OT complex; in case of going out of OT complex entire attire should be changed until or unless OT personnel comes back to OT complex.

Explanation

According to Centers for Disease Control and Prevention (CDC) guidelines[15] use of surgical mask helps to prevent a mechanical barrier for oropharyngeal and nasopharyngeal secretions. Surgical attire fabrics should be tightly woven, stain resistant and durable. Fabric pores should be less than 80 microns otherwise it may allow microorganisms attached to skin squamous to pass through the interstices of the material's weave. Tightly woven surgical attire reduces the amount of bacteria shed into the air by two to five times, with the exception of Methicillin-resistant *Staphylococcus epidermidis* (MRSE) from MRSE carriers.[16] OT attire should be resistant to punctures and tears to prevent microbial contamination of the sterile field. It should be impervious and fluid-resistant to prevent strike-through contamination from microorganisms. OT attire should be lint free as lint is recognized as a vector for causing surgical site infection (SSI).

Should OT personnel be screened for infective focus?

We recommend that MRSA screening is required for healthcare workers at the time of job joining and then yearly. If an OT personnel have to undergo any surgical intervention on him/her or visits any other hospital; then we need to screen OT personnel again for MRSA. Nasal swabs can be used for screening of MRSA carriers.

Explanation

The MRSA circulated in hospital among patients, healthcare workers and the environment. The timing and cost-effectiveness of screening and decolonization of healthcare workers with MRSA nasal carriage deserves further attention. Screening and decolonization treatment in combination with hand hygiene eliminated the cross transmission between patients, healthcare workers and the environment. It is important to screen healthcare workers at the time of joining.[17]

What are recovery room protocols?

The recovery suite should be in a central position within the theater complex enabling ease of access from the OT, but with a separate outside access for transfer of patients to the ward. Size of a recovery room facility to the number of OT served, e.g., a recovery area of 164 m^2 for a department of eight theaters. The ratio of beds to operating theaters should not be less than two. The beds should allow unobstructed access for trolleys, X-ray equipment, resuscitation carts and clinical staff. The facility should be open plan allowing each recovery area to be observed, but with the provision of curtains for optional patient privacy. To keep the area sterile and prevent the spreading of germs, outside visitors may be required to use a gown and cap or may be prohibited completely. Patients must be observed on a one-to-one basis by an anesthetist, recovery nurse or other properly trained member of staff until they have regained airway control and cardiovascular stability and are able to communicate. This helps to minimize postoperative complication.

SUMMARY

1. Operation theater personal should follow strict hand hygiene rules and use alcohol-based hand rubs. Wearing of gloves is essential while cleaning or handling equipment.
2. Operation theater traffic should be kept minimum and strict rules and regulations along with proper training and education of the staff is needed.
3. Operation theater attire should not be worn outside the OT complex. In case OT attire is used outside the OT, it should be changed once the personnel return to OT.
4. Methicillin-resistant *Staphylococcus aureus* screening should be done at the time of joining and then yearly thereafter for all OT personnel.

REFERENCES

1. Centers for disease control and prevention (2007). Guidelines for isolation precautions: preventing translation of infectious agents in healthcare settings. [online]. Available from http://www.cdc.gov/hicpac/2007ip_table.html [Accessed June 6, 2014].
2. Boyce JM, Opal SM, Chow JW, et al. Outbreak of multidrug-resistant Enterococcus faecium with transferable vanB class vancomycin resistance. J Clin Microbiol. 1994;32(5):1148-53.
3. Krediet AC, Kalkman CJ, Bonten MJ, et al. Hand-hygiene practices in the operating theatre: an observational study. Br J Anaesth. 2011;107(4):553-8.
4. Widmer AF, Rotter M. Effectiveness of alcohol-based hand hygiene gels in reducing nosocomial infection rate. Infect Control Hosp Epidemiol. 2008;29(6):576.
5. Pittet D, Hugonnet S, Harbarth S, et al. Effectiveness of a hospital-wide programme to improve compliance with hand hygiene. Infection Control Programme. Lancet. 2000;356(9238):1307-12.
6. Al-Maiyah M, Bajwa A, Mackenney P, et al. Glove perforation and contamination in primary total hip arthroplasty. J Bone Joint Surg Br. 2005;87(4):556-9.

7. Beldame J, Lagrave B, Leivain L, et al. Surgical glove bacterial contamination and perforation during total hip arthroplasty implantation: when gloves should be changed. Orthop Traumatol Surg Res. 2012;98(4):432-40.
8. Kaya I, Ugras A, Sungur I, et al. Glove perforation time and frequency in total hip arthroplasty procedures. Acta Orthop Traumatol Turc. 2012;46(1):57-60.
9. Laine T, Aarnio P. How often does glove perforation occur in surgery? Comparison between single gloves and a double-gloving system. Am J Surg. 2001;181(6):564-6.
10. Ritter MA, Eitzen H, Franch ML, et al. The operating room environment as affected by people and the surgical face mask. Clin Orthop Relat Res. 1975;111:147-50.
11. Panahi P, Stroh M, Casper DS, et al. Operating room traffic is a major concern during total joint arthroplasty. Clin Orthop Relat Res. 2012;470(10):2690-4.
12. Andersson AE, Bergh I, Karlsson J, et al. Traffic flow in the operating room: an explorative and descriptive study on air quality during orthopedic trauma implant surgery. Am J Infect Control. 2012;40(8):750-5.
13. Allo MD, Tedesco M. Operating room management: operative suite considerations, infection control. Surg Clin North Am. 2005;85(6):1291-7.
14. Lynch RJ, Englesbe MJ, Sturm L, et al. Measurement of foot traffic in the operating room: implications for infection control. Am J Med Qual. 2009;24(1):45-52.
15. Mangram AJ, Horan TC, Pearson ML, et al. Guideline for Prevention of Surgical Site Infection, 1999. Centers for Disease Control and Prevention (CDC) Hospital Infection Control Practices Advisory Committee. Am J Infect Control. 1999;27(2):97-132.
16. Perioperative Standards and Recommended Practices. [online]. Available from http://www.aornstandards.org/content/1/SEC4.extract [Accessed June 19, 2014].
17. Blok HE, Troelstra A, Kamp-Hopmans TE, et al. "Role of healthcare workers in outbreaks of methicillin-resistant Staphylococcus aureus: a 10-year evaluation from a Dutch university hospital. Infection Control and Hospital Epidemiology. 2003;24(9): 679-85.

Section 2

Perioperative Patient Preparation

Section Outline

6. Patient Optimization
7. Patient and Operative Site Preparation
8. Intraoperative Protocols
9. Postoperative Management
10. Prophylactic Antibiotics

6

Patient Optimization

*Aditi Malpani, Himanshu Dongre,
Bharati Adhye, Pramod P Neema, Ashok Shyam*

INTRODUCTION

Preoperatively, it is essential to evaluate patients for pre-existing medical conditions followed by optimization of comorbidities. Patients should be assessed for presence of risk factors and susceptibility to infection. Specific risk factors such as the following are to be identified before surgery can be categorized as below:

- Physiological risk factors like associated anatomical abnormalities, autoimmune disorders, immunodeficiency disorders, etc.
- Comorbidities like hypertension, diabetes mellitus (DM), asthma, cardiac issues, allergies or treatments like chemotherapy, dialysis, radiation, etc.
- Personal factors like poor hygiene, prolonged immobility, etc.
- Associated diseases that have high risk of transmission like tuberculosis (TB), hepatitis B, human immunodeficiency virus (HIV), etc.
- Pediatric patients and elderly patients need additional assessment.

Patient education is a vital component in preventing surgical site infection (SSI). In this chapter, following comorbidities affecting SSI will be discussed in details:

- Diabetes
- Autoimmune disorders

- HIV and hepatitis B
- Systemic skin diseases like psoriasis
- Hematological disorders like sickle cell disease
- Asthma
- Chronic kidney disease (CKD).

What is the optimization protocol for patients with diabetes?

Diabetes is the major risk factor for postoperative wound complications. All patients undergoing surgery should be screened for diabetes preoperatively. Fasting blood sugar level and urine ketones should be checked on the day of surgery. In elective surgeries, HbA1c levels should be optimized to less than 7%. In patients with HbA1c between 7% and 8%, should be subjected to surgery considering merit of the particular case. Elective cases should be postponed till optimization, if HbA1c levels are more than 7%. In emergency and trauma cases, random blood sugar level should be optimized to less than 200 mg%.

Explanation

Perioperative hyperglycemia is independently associated with surgical wound complications.[1,2] Wound infection has been shown to be more common in patients with diabetes after surgery and in non-diabetic patients who developed transient postoperative hyperglycemia.[3] Hyperglycemia is associated with increased monocyte susceptibility to apoptosis and impaired neutrophil function. In various studies, the investigators have concluded that patients with a mean perioperative blood glucose of > 200 mg/dL or preoperative HbA1c levels of > 6.7% are at increased risk for wound complications following elective primary total joint arthroplasty.[4,5] In a retrospective study of 167 total knee replacement patients, it was found that independent risk factor for wound complications was preoperative HbA1c more than 8%.

These inferences are based on numerous studies specifically in areas of joint arthroplasty,[6,7] but also in spine surgery and trauma surgeries where increased risk of surgery has been found with poor glycemic control. Olsen et al studied the risk factors for surgical site infection following orthopedic spinal operations.[8] Jan and Richards et al studied the relationship of hyperglycemia and SSI in orthopedic surgery.[9] In trauma cases, Karunakar and Staples showed that mean perioperative glucose levels >220 mg/dL [hyperglycemic index (HGI) >3.0] were associated with a seven times higher risk of infection in orthopedic trauma patients with not known history of diabetes mellitus.[10] These may be defined as having stress-induced hyperglycemia rather than diabetic hyperglycemia. Stress hyperglycemia and SSI in stable non-diabetic adults with orthopedic injuries. Kerby et al stated that stress-induced hyperglycemia, not diabetic hyperglycemia, is associated with higher mortality in trauma.[11] However, definitive works and quantification is still awaited. It would be advisable to do an HbAc1 test in these patients to diagnose occult diabetes (Hb1Ac levels > 6.5 with random blood sugar levels > 200 mg%). These patients would need a proper and continued diabetic care postoperatively.

What is the optimization protocol for hypertensive patients?

The potential benefits of delaying surgery to optimize the effects of anti-hypertensive medications should be weighed against the risk of delaying the surgical procedure. Anti-hypertensives should be continued in the perioperative period. Angiotensin-converting enzyme (ACE) inhibitors may be required to be stopped and replaced by short-acting anti-hypertensives, till the patient is euvolemic again. In emergency cases, rapid-acting intravenous anti-hypertensives may control the blood pressure (BP) in matter of hours and surgery can be performed with due risk.

> **Explanation**

Although hypertension is not in itself an independent risk factor for SSI; however, associated comorbidities and medication may increase the risk of delayed wound healing.[12] Stopping of anti-hypertensives may cause intraoperative hypertensive crises and cardiovascular complications. Patients should be maintained on their regular antihypertensives throughout the preoperative period. Oral dose should be given on the morning of surgery, with parental control till the patient is able to take oral medication. ACE inhibitors have been shown to cause intraoperative hypovolemia and renal problems in perioperative period due to fluctuations in the blood volume and thus are recommended to discontinue before surgery. They can be restarted once the euvolemic status has been achieved.[13]

Associated medications are discussed along with cardiac diseases subsequently later in this chapter.

What is the optimization protocol for patients with autoimmune disorders?

Obtaining drug history and examining for presence of any organ dysfunction or active skin lesions in all patients with autoimmune disorders like rheumatoid arthritis (RA), systemic lupus erythematosus (SLE), ankylosing spondylitis is essential. Steroids need to be titrated as per risk/benefit ratio and patient on long-term steroids (or steroid-dependent disease control) will require perioperative steroids. Disease-modifying antirheumatic drugs (DMARDs) do not increase infection rate and need not be stopped before surgery. Anti-tumor necrosis factor (TNF) therapy has to be balanced on a risk benefit scale, as it is still debatable if they significantly increase the risk of infection. However, it is safer to stop biologic therapy before undergoing elective surgeries.

Explanation

Rheumatoid arthritis is an independent risk factor for infection in arthroplasty.[14,15] There is high incidence and subsequent reinfection, as these patients often present for arthroplasty early in life.

Local and systemic corticosteroids have been shown to delay wound healing, increase the risk of wound infection and cause adrenal insufficiency. Continuation of steroid should be titrated as per risk and benefit in individual cases. In patients who are steroid dependent have to be continued on perioperative steroids and surgical team should be ready for any eventual complications. The British Society for Rheumatology (BSR) guidelines suggest that in most cases, disease-modifying antirheumatic drugs (DMARDs) should not be stopped before joint replacement. Methotrexate (MTX) is a commonly used first-line drug and is not considered to increase wound infection risk, and should not be discontinued before orthopedic surgery.[16-19] TNF-α is an inflammatory cytokine (highly concentrated in the synovial tissue of RA patients) implicated in joint destruction. Any increase in risk of infection in patients who received anti-TNF therapy before surgery is debatable. The BSR guidelines 2010 state that the potential benefit of preventing postoperative infections (by stopping treatment) should be balanced against the risk of a perioperative disease flare. If anti-TNF therapy is to be withheld, it should be discontinued between 5 and 20 days before surgery (three to five times the half-life of the drug), restarting when there is good wound healing and no evidence of infection (1 week for Enbrel, 6–8 weeks for Remicade and 2 weeks for Humira). Majority of evidence is based around the use of MTX in the perioperative period. Based on trial data and clinical experience, the consensus in the United Kingdom is that treatment with MTX should not be stopped in patients whose disease is controlled prior to elective orthopedic procedures. The current best evidence for this is the prospective randomized controlled trial by Grennan et al[16] that involved 388 patients with RA and suggested that there was no increased risk of infection or other postoperative complications in patients with RA who continued MTX. However, in elderly frail patients with comorbidities and a degree of renal impairment, it may be prudent to withhold MTX the week prior to surgery, as MTX is renally excreted. MTX should be reinstated as soon as the patient is stable postoperatively. For the remaining DMARDs in current use, the available data does not support any clear evidence-based recommendations.

What is the optimization protocol for HIV and hepatitis B?

Preoperative CD4, CD8 levels and HIV viral load should be done within 1 week prior to the surgery. CD4 counts should be more than 350 cells/μL, CD8 count should be more than 100 cells/mcL, CD4:CD8 ratio should be more than 2 and viral load should be less than 30,000 copies per milliliter. In emergency trauma cases, we can perform surgery with low CD4 count, but a prolonged antibiotic coverage will be needed.

In case of hepatitis B positive patients, liver function tests, serum electrolytes, sugar level, prothrombin time, BT-CT, HBsAg and HBeAg, anti-HBe, anti-HBs status should be checked. Ultrasonography of abdomen should be done preoperative for presence of cirrhosis, ascites and signs of portal hypertension. Neurological signs—encephalopathy should be determined.

Explanation

In the HIV-positive population, concern exists that impaired immune defense to common and uncommon surgical pathogens may lead to delayed wound healing and osteoarticular infection. There is paucity of literature comparing surgical outcome, healthy individuals and HIV infected patients. In a multicenter observational study, SSI rate was two-fold higher than that reported for the general population, with more severe clinical presentations.[20] According to guidelines given by New York State Department of health AIDS institute, particularly the presence or absence of organ failure and nutritional status (albumin less than 2.5 g/dL) have been found to be more reliable predictors of surgical outcome than CD4 count or viral load in HIV infected patients.[21] Poor surgical results in terms of SSI have been reported in some studies where CD4 count was low (< 300 cells/µL).[22] Another prospective study by Howard et al does not support the hypothesis that HIV infection per se increases postoperative SSI and suggested that treatment of fractures should not be altered in HIV positive patients with CD4 counts > 350 cells/µL.[23] Preoperative CD4 levels done within 1 week of the surgery should be considered. Patients with CD4 counts < 350 cells/µL, elective surgeries should defer till optimal levels of CD4 counts are achieved.

Associated comorbidities that are more prevalent in the HIV infected population should be optimized:
- Hepatic and renal dysfunction
- Coronary artery disease
- Coagulopathy, thrombocytopenia and neutropenia
- Active alcohol or substance use
- History of prior infection/colonization with methicillin-resistant *Staphylococcus aureus* (should receive vancomycin instead of cefazolin for prophylaxis when indicated)
- Drug allergies and drug interactions (protease inhibitors may cause severe interactions; midazolam is contraindicated in combination with ritonavir).

HIV infected patients should be mobilized postoperatively as soon as medically feasible because of increased risk of thromboembolic complications. A survey conducted by Kigera et al[24] noted that there is increased risk of 1.8 times with patient having HIV, but studies are poorly constructed and there were small sample. In trauma study by Guild et al[25] shows CD4 count is associated with postoperative infection in patients with orthopedic trauma who are HIV positive. In these cases either we wait for CD count to rise or perform surgery under prolonged antibiotic coverage.

Patients with chronic hepatitis without evidence of cirrhosis or hepatic decompensation generally do not have an increased complication risk. Patients with decompensated cirrhosis (child's class C), acute alcoholic hepatitis and acute viral hepatitis, and patients with evidence of hepatic decompensation (hypoalbuminemia, coagulopathy, ascites and encephalopathy) carry a high risk of perioperative complications and early prosthetic failure risk. Infection is a common cause of failure and may be difficult to treat.[26]

What is the optimization protocol for systemic skin diseases like psoriasis?

Active lesions in and around surgical site can increase risk of infection. Routine preoperative skin preparation and the usual perioperative antibiotics are adequate for the prevention of infection in the psoriatic patient. However, attempt should be made to achieve the best possible control of psoriatic lesions in the vicinity of an elective incision. Prior consultation with dermatologist should be sought. For compound fracture, 5 days antibiotic regimen should be considered. As far as possible, the psoriatic lesion site is to be avoided.

Explanation

Psoriasis is an autoimmune disease for which the treatment revolves around the use of corticosteroids and immunomodulators. These drugs are already discussed above and same precautions are to be taken in cases with psoriasis.

Along with these therapeutic considerations, psoriasis itself is an independent risk factor for postoperative infection.[27]

What is the optimization protocol for hematological diseases like sickle cell disease?

In patients suffering from sickle cell disease, there can be increased risk of postoperative infection due to autosplenectomy. Associated presence of pneumonitis, osteomyelitis can act as source of infection. Potential complications include postoperative hemorrhage, wound hematoma requiring evacuation, dislocated prosthesis and wound infection with abscess formation (10–20%). We suggest considering transfusion to build up hemoglobin level to 10 g/dL and HbS% to be less than 30%.

Hydroxyurea should be started or more months preoperative for patients with more than three sickle crises per year (requiring admission to hospital or severe vaso-occlusive complications). Hydroxyurea has been used in chemotherapy, but has been found quite effective in reducing the frequency and severity of sickle crisis. It works by increasing the production of fetal hemoglobin (HbF) which are resistant to sickling, thus lowering the HbS concentration and preventing sickling complications. Aggressive remobilization should be aimed at in postoperative period to prevent thromboembolic complications and atelectasis. Thromboembolism prophylaxis with low-molecular-weight heparin (LMWH) is indicated. It trigger factors for sickling crisis like dehydration, fever and pain, and thus should be avoided.

Explanation

The most common pre-existing condition is pulmonary disease (previous episode of acute chest syndrome or chronic lung disease), followed by central nervous system disease (cerebral vascular accident, cerebral palsy and isolated seizure disorder). *Streptococcus pneumoniae* infection is one of the major causes of morbidity in cases of sickle cell disease.[28] The cause of increased risk of infection include immunoparesis secondary to autosplenectomy, compromised blood flow associated with poor antibiotic delivery to the tissues and prolonged surgical time.

Hemoglobin value, HbS%, renal function tests, liver function tests, reticulocyte count, and serum LDH levels should be checked. Chest X-ray, pulmonary function tests (PFTs), arterial blood gas (ABG), and electrocardiogram (ECG) should be done before surgery. Preoperative transfusion results in enhanced oxygen-carrying capacity of the erythrocytes. This facilitates an increase in overall microvascular perfusion, which is associated with a decrease in the risk of postoperative sickle cell crises. The decision of transfusion depends not only on the hemoglobin level but also the clinical status, pattern and severity of sickle exacerbations, presence of organ damage and symptomatic anemia (symptoms of myocardial ischemia, orthostatic hypotension or tachycardia unresponsive to fluid replacement). Transfusion itself has its own complications like development of new red cell antibodies and hemolytic transfusion reactions. Thus, risk and benefits of transfusion in cases of sickle cell anemia (SCA) with trauma should be carefully weighted and probably a less aggressive strategy of maintaining the Hb levels to 10 mg% (as opposed to more aggressive strategy of reducing HbS level to < 30%) would be more optimal in these trauma cases.[29]

What is the optimization protocol for asthma?

Rates of pulmonary complications are increased in cases where asthma is uncontrolled. In these patients, the pulmonary function tests are altered and with FEV1 and FVC < 70%, FEV1/FVC ratio < 65%, there is high risk of postoperative pulmonary complications.[30] It can also lead to increased postoperative infection rates. Bronchodilators, in selected patients (those on systemic steroids within the last 6 months) intravenous steroids, antibiotics, and smoking cessation can all help to reduce complications. In case of smokers, 8 weeks is the optimum period for cessation in order to prevent complications associated with smoking.

Explanation

Association of Chest Physicians (ACPs) consensus statement recommends preoperative pulmonary function test (PFT) in patients undergoing arthroplasty with unexplained dyspnea and pulmonary symptoms. In controlled asthmatics, a short-acting β2 agonist is added just prior to surgery. In moderately controlled patients, inhaled corticosteroids such as beclomethasone 400 µg is added to their β2 agonist's treatment 1 week prior to surgery. Poorly controlled asthmatics may need to add oral corticosteroids to their regimen. Studies confirm the safety of perioperative systemic corticosteroids surgery. Methylprednisolone or hydrocortisone 100 mg intravenously every 8 hours should be started the morning before surgery.

A study done by Kaye et al concluded that chronic obstructive pulmonary disease (COPD) is an independent risk factor in elderly patients undergoing spinal surgery.[31] Another study done by Koutsoumbelis et al identified COPD as a risk factor for postoperative infection following posterior spinal instrumentation for fusion.[32]

What is the optimization protocol for chronic kidney disease (CKD)?

Meticulous aseptic precautions and judicial use of non-nephrotoxic broad-spectrum antibiotics should be used in patients with chronic renal disease. Optimization of the patient with renal dysfunction needs not only to consider the pre-existing renal functions but also the potential risk of acute kidney injury in the perioperative setting. CKD patients on dialysis, having invasive lines and those with presence of complications due to chronic renal failure, have increased susceptibility to postoperative infections.[33]

The incidence and severity of acute renal failure usually is greater when preoperative serum creatinine level is > 2 mg/dL. Up to creatinine level 2, the patient can be subjected to surgery. If creatinine levels are > 2, nephrologist's opinion should be sought.

Explanation

Bohenski et al performed a longitudinal retrospective cohort study and found that chronic renal disease is one of the important factor for postoperative complications including deep vein thrombosis (DVT) and SSI.[34] In a retrospective analytical study by Miric et al inferred that CKD patients undergoing knee replacements have more comorbidities and a higher risk for superficial SSI, 90-day readmission and anytime mortality.[35] Overall, the risk of developing postoperative infection after total joint arthroplasty is significantly higher in patients with chronic renal failure, especially in those on hemodialysis. Hence, we recommend that patients with CKD may have received multiple transfusions and they can develop antibodies that can significantly delay processing for packed red blood cells. Electrolyte disturbances are common and hyperkalemia is a frequent concern.

What modifications in antiplatelet drugs should be done before surgery? Also what regimens are required in patients with coronary artery bypass grafting (CABG), postangioplasty, intracardiac devices in situ and cerebrovascular accidents?

We recommend that if the patient is on dual antiplatelet therapy (aspirin and clopidogrel), then modification of the therapy should be based on weighing the risk of thrombosis verses risk of perioperative bleeding. In patients with high risk for bleeding and low risk for ischemic events, aspirin should be continued (low dose, i.e., 75 mg) and clopidogrel should be stopped for 5–7 days preoperative and restarted 48 hours postoperative. Dual antiplatelet therapy should be continued when there is low-bleeding risk. Patients with coronary stents in situ have a high thrombotic risk if antiplatelet drug therapy is interrupted. Elective non-cardiac surgery should therefore be avoided after stent placement, i.e., during the first 6 weeks for bare metal stents and during the first 12 months for drug-eluting stents (DES).[36,37]

Explanation

In a systematic review on joint replacement surgeries, the investigators realized that perioperative management of patients with cardiac diseases in receipt of antithrombotic agents is based upon a delicate balance between the perceived risk of arterial thromboembolism and the perceived risk of perioperative bleeding.[38]

Patients who are at high risk of thrombotic events include those with any mechanical heart valve, atrial fibrillation with history of stroke or transient ischemic attack or rheumatic valvular heart disease, recent venous thromboembolism (within 3 months), and recurring venous thromboembolism receiving long-term anticoagulation.[39,40]

The ACC/AHA guidelines state that if clopidogrel has been stopped preoperatively, then serious consideration should be given for continuation of aspirin preoperatively. As per the guidelines of Society of Thoracic Surgeons (2012), stopping clopidogrel for 5–7 days before surgery does not have any adverse effect on cardiovascular function, but it decreases intraoperative bleeding.

An increase in bleeding complications is well recognized with the combination of aspirin and clopidogrel compared with aspirin alone in both medical and surgical patients. Excess bleeding in surgical patients could increase the risk of infection by increasing the need for blood transfusion or surgical re-exploration.[41–43] In emergency (trauma), patients need to be assessed on a case-by-case basis. In situations where the risk of intraoperative bleeding in patients taking clopidogrel is less than the morbidity/mortality of delaying treatment, (e.g. fractured neck of femur[16–18]), surgery should not be delayed. Surgeons should be aware of the mechanism of action of clopidogrel and its potential side effects, and surgical technique should be modified accordingly.[44]

What is the role of preoperative oropharyngeal check-up and what should be the timing of dental procedures in the perioperative period?

All patients undergoing elective surgeries should be screened for presence of oropharyngeal infections. Also signs and symptoms of active dental infection (cavities, periodontal abscesses and severe gingivitis) should be checked. History of recent dental procedures should be determined. Except for cases of trauma; joint replacement surgery can usually be delayed until 4–6 weeks after periodontal treatment. Also no dental procedure should be undertaken for at least 6–8 weeks after the surgery.

Explanation

Postoperative prosthetic joint infections are uncommon and occur at a rate of 1–2%. Bacteremia by both aerobic and anaerobic organisms can occur as a result of dental treatment particularly during extraction of erupted, periodontal involved teeth.[45] Transient bacteremia may occur spontaneously without any dental treatment. Late infections have been observed with *Streptococcus viridians* in patients with poor oral health without any dental procedures. This study implicates an oral origin for infection rather than formal dental manipulation, which perhaps emphasizes the need for good oral hygiene prior to and after arthroplasty surgery.[46] For the first postoperative year, antibiotic prophylaxis is recommended prior to all dental manipulations except routine cleanings. After the 1st year, antibiotic prophylaxis is required only for 'high-risk' procedures, such as extraction or root canal that cause bleeding.[47]

What is the significance of routine preoperative urine screening?

Urinary tract infection can create reservoir of pathogens that can increase risk of postoperative wound infections.[48,49] Urine microscopy should be < 8 pus cells/hpf before posting patient for elective arthroplasty.

Explanation

Routine preoperative urine screening should be done in all surgeries (elective and trauma) and should be accompanied by urine cultures if microscopy shows > 8 pus cells/hpf. Patients can be asymptomatic in spite of positive culture reports. These have higher risk of postoperative wound complications.[50–52] Patients should be started on antibiotics preoperative if symptomatic or if culture reports are positive.

How do smoking and alcohol consumption increase rate of postoperative infection?

Smoking and alcohol consumption are associated with postoperative morbidity (delayed wound healing, infections, and longer hospital stay) and mortality. Current smoking (at the time of elective surgeries) is associated with increased risk of pneumonia and SSIs.

Explanation

Patients consuming alcohol daily have significant increased risk of postoperative infections after arthroplasty.[53,54] Alcohol elevates the levels of cortisol and interleukin-10 that impair proper functioning of the immune system. It prolongs bleeding time and increases risk of bleeding during and after surgery. Acute ethanol exposure can lead to impaired wound healing by impairing the early inflammatory response, inhibiting wound closure, angiogenesis, and collagen production, and altering the protease balance at the wound site. Chronic alcohol exposure causes impaired wound healing and enhanced host susceptibility to infections. Abstinence starting 3–8 weeks before surgery will significantly reduce the incidence of postoperative wound and cardiopulmonary complications and infections.

Smoking causes temporary reduction in tissue perfusion and oxygenation, impaired inflammatory cell function, oxidative bactericidal mechanisms and attenuation of reparative cell function. In smokers, postoperative healing complications and nonunions occur more as compared to nonsmoker. Current smoking at the time of total hip replacement (THR) or total knee replacement (TKR) is associated with increased risk of SSI.[55–57] Smokers have been shown to suffer higher rates of flap failure, tissue necrosis and hematoma formation. If microvascular surgery is to be performed, persistent smoking significantly increases the rate of postoperative complications, with wound infection due to constriction of peripheral microvasculature.

What is the significance of perioperative blood transfusions with respect to postoperative infection rates?

Blood transfusions are associated with increased risk of postoperative wound infections. More the number of units given and older the blood increase the risk of infection. However, transfusion may be necessary in cases where preoperative Hb is below 10 mg% (in emergency cases, this cut off can be < 9 mg% with careful calibration of blood loss and replacements).

Risks include:
- **Transfusion transmitted infections:** Viral infections—human immunodeficiency virus (HIV) 1:1,000,000; hepatitis B virus (HBV) 1:100,000; hepatitis C virus (HCV) 1:500–1:5,000; human T-lymphocytic virus 1 and 2 (HTLV) 1:200,000; cytomegalovirus (CMV) 1:2,500; bacterial infections 1:400,000 transfusions and Creutzfeldt-Jakob disease.
- **Direct immune injury:** Mild hemolytic reactions range from 1:5,000 to severe hemolytic reactions and anaphylaxis in 1:600,000.
- **Immunomodulation:** In vitro, allogeneic blood has been shown to have the capacity to depress immune function mediated mainly by transfused white blood cells.
- **Procedural/Clerical error:** Serious complications include coagulopathy, renal failure, intravascular hemolysis, persistent viral infection and death.

Explanation

Blood transfusion can increase risk of infection in both elective and trauma orthopedic procedures.[58,59] Minimizing the use of old blood, stored for more than 15 days may decrease the risk of postoperative complications including infection. Allogeneic blood products have immunomodulatory effects that may increase the risk of nosocomial infections. It is also possible that the transfusion of blood products act as a marker for individuals with a greater number of comorbidities and other SSI risk factors, which independently places them at an inherently greater risk of infection. *Staphylococcus aureus* was found to be the cause of most of the infections (41%), followed by *Staphylococcus epidermidis* (16.4%) and *Enterococcus*.[51] In a study, infection rate of 27% as opposed to 15% in transfused versus non-transfused patients undergoing open reduction and internal fixation for hip fracture was seen. Similarly, infection rate of 7% in patients who were transfused versus 3% in non-transfused patients was noted in a study undergoing elective joint arthroplasty.

What are the criteria for optimal nutritional status with regards to optimization before surgery?

Undernutrition as well as obesity both can increase the risk of SSI. Nutritional status of patients should be assessed prior to surgery by subjective assessment (dietary intake, gastrointestinal symptoms, etc.) and by laboratory parameters, which ideally should be hemoglobin level > 10 g/dL, serum albumin > 3 g/dL, CRP < 10 mg/dL. Increased body mass index (BMI), body fat percentage (BF%), independent risk factors for SSI, and additional precautions are warranted when operating on patients with high BMI and BF%.

Explanation

Malnutrition

Malnutrition has five to seven-fold higher risk of developing major wound complications. Patients are at greater risk of prolonged hospital stay.[60,61] In 2008, there was a study showing an increased risk of infection in total joint arthroplasty based on socioeconomic background.[53]

Malnutrition can be diagnosed if the serum transferrin level is < 200 mg/dL, the serum albumin is < 3.5 g/dL and the total lymphocyte count is < 1,800 cells/cumm. Other parameters include CRP, anemia, prealbumin < 16 mg/dL, vitamin deficiency, involuntary weight loss >10%.

Presence of pedal edema, facial swelling, ascites, muscle wasting and loss of subcutaneous fat, all these indicate undernutrition. Preoperative serum albumin status is the strong predictor of complications within first 30 days postoperative.

Obesity

Obese patients have significantly higher risk of postoperative complications, such as wound infection.[62,63] Morbidly obese patients with diabetes had the highest rate of infection, with 5 out of 51 patients (9.8%) developing infection.[64] Increased length and complexity of surgery and poorer vascularization of the subcutaneous layer may contribute to this elevated risk. Obese patients also require a significantly higher fraction of inspired oxygen (FIO2) to reach an adequate arterial oxygen level. Dose of antibiotics also need to be adjusted as per the body weight. Few short-term studies have shown compared to primary THA, revision surgery in obese patients is a longer and more complicated procedure implying more extensive tissue damage, and a greater risk of prosthetic joint infections and dislocation.[65-69]

Are the elderly more prone to infection?

The elderly are prone to infections during their hospital stay preoperatively as well as postoperatively. Reduced immune responses, poor nutrition, comorbidities, ongoing medications, all these factors pose risk increasing susceptibility to infections. We recommend preoperative optimization of all comorbidities before surgery, antibiotic prophylaxis where indicated, nutritional supplementation, aggressive control of blood glucose levels, maintenance of core body temperature and adequate oxygenation.

Explanation

Surgical site infections (SSIs) account for approximately 11% of the nosocomial infections among the older patients.[70] There are risk factors associated with senescence itself and there are diseases that predispose patients to infection and are found with increased prevalence among elderly patients.[71] Systemic oxygenation is necessary to maintain adequate levels of tissue oxygenation at the skin. Greif et al demonstrated a reduction in the rate of SSI (from 11.2% to 5.2%) among patients who were maintained on supranormal oxygen levels. Although the effect of supranormal oxygenation remains unclear, frank hypoxia should be rigorously avoided. The nutritional status of elderly patients too influences postoperative recovery. Early diagnosis of infections is essential, given that morbidity and mortality have significant roles in such conditions. The atypical presentation of some manifestations of infections constitutes a further challenge. It is known that only 60% of elderly individuals with severe infectious conditions develop leukocytosis; also in this regard, the response to fever may be weak and temperature greater than 38.3°C may indicate severe infection. Pneumonia, urinary infections and skin infections occur frequently. Another risk factor is admission from a healthcare facility.[72] Elderly patients with SSI have worse outcomes than do younger patients. The difference is probably related to diminished host response.

How do systemic foci of infection affect postoperative infection rates?

In patients with systemic foci of infection, especially upper respiratory tract infection and urinary tract infection, there is high chances of developing SSI and increased overall morbidity. Hence, RTI should be treated completely before elective surgery. In emergency cases, these foci should be aggressively treated simultaneously and patient need to be communicated about high risk of infection and possibility of longer or stronger antibiotics.

In patients suffering from tuberculosis, liver function tests LFTs, PFTs and ABG should be done. Antituberculous agents are continued on the day of surgery to keep blood levels constant and may be administered with a small amount of water. Patient wears a mask when leaving the room.

Explanation

Staphylococcus aureus is the main microbial pathogen in orthopedic infections. The infection caused by *S. aureus* is attributable to patients' endogenous colonization. The ecologic niche of *S. aureus* is the anterior nares and nasal carriage increases the risk of the development of a SSI.[73] If the patient has active infection, this infection can cause pneumonia postoperatively and would increase morbidity. Despite this, the presence of a upper respiratory infection (URI) does not appear to affect the patient's overall length of hospital stay nor the development of long-term sequelae.[74-77] Hence, further prospective studies are required to specifically state that elective surgery should be postponed in view of active URI.

Droplet nuclei can be dispersed widely by air currents and remain suspended in the air for a long period, which can affect a large number of patients and staff members; therefore, airborne precautions must be instituted. Patients with TB may have an inability to clear secretions or obstructions from the respiratory tract to maintain a clear airway and may have pneumonia as a result of retained secretions. Patients with TB may also have an ineffective cough as a result of malnutrition and weakness.

SUMMARY

1. In patients with diabetes, the HbA1c should be optimized to be below 7% for elective surgery. In case of an emergency surgery, random blood sugar should be optimized to be less than 200 mg%.
2. In hypertensives, the elective surgeries can be performed in diastolic blood pressure < 110 mm Hg. For emergency cases, risk assessment should be done and in case surgery cannot be delayed, BP can be controlled by using rapid-acting intravenous agents. ACE inhibitors have to be withheld in perioperative period, while all other antihypertensive agents should be continued throughout the perioperative period.

3. In rheumatoid disorders, DMARDs should be continued, while biological therapeutics should be discontinued. Steroids need to be titrated as per the risk benefit ratio and should be continued in cases, which are steroid dependent.
4. For specific diseases like HIV, hepatitis, sickle cell disease and asthma, individualized protocols of investigation and management would be required for optimization.
5. For patients on antiplatelet therapy, the bleeding versus thromboembolism risks have to be assessed.
6. Smoking and drinking should be stopped around 5–8 weeks before elective surgery.
7. Nutritional status including the hemoglobin levels need to be optimized in all elective cases.

For the sake of simplicity, this chapter has compartmentalized the patient optimization into individual diseases or situations. However, many patients present with multiple comorbidities and individualized approach to optimizing them is essential.

REFERENCES

1. Hyuk Soo Han, Seung-Baik Kang. Relations between long-term glycemic control and postoperative wound and infectious complications after total knee arthroplasty in type 2 diabetics. Clin Orthop Surg. 2013;5(2):118-23.
2. Subramaniam B, Lerner A, Novack V, et al. Increased glycemic variability in patients with elevated preoperative HbA1C predicts adverse outcomes following coronary artery bypass grafting surgery. Anesth Analg. 2014;118(2):277-87.
3. Stryker LS, Abdel MP, Morrey ME, et al. Elevated postoperative blood glucose and preoperative hemoglobin A1C are associated with increased wound complications following total joint arthroplasty. J Bone Joint Surg Am. 2013;95(9):808-14, S1-2.
4. Tennyson C, Lee R, Attia R. Is there a role for HbA1c in predicting mortality and morbidity outcomes after coronary artery bypass graft surgery? Interact Cardiovasc Thorac Surg. 2013;17(6): 1000-8.
5. Louis S Stryker, Matthew P Abdel, Mark E Morrey, et al. Elevated postoperative blood glucose and preoperative hemoglobin A1C

are associated with increased wound complications following total joint arthroplasty. J Bone Joint Surg Am. 2013;95(9):808-14.
6. Iorio R, Williams KM, Marcantonio AJ, et al. Diabetes mellitus, hemoglobin A1C and the incidence of total joint arthroplasty infection. Journal of Arthroplasty. 2012;27(5):726-9.
7. Adams AL, Paxton EW, Wang JQ, et al. Surgical outcomes of total knee replacement according to diabetes status and glycemic control, 2001 to 2009. J Bone Joint Surg Am. 2013;95 (6):481-7.
8. Olsen MA, Nepple JJ, Riew KD, et al. Risk factors for surgical site infection following orthopaedic spinal operations. J Bone Joint Surg Am. 2008;90(1):62-9.
9. Richards JE, Kauffmann RM, Zuckerman SL, et al. Relationship of hyperglycemia and surgical-site infection in orthopaedic surgery. J Bone Joint Surg Am 2012;94(13):1181-6.
10. Pull ter Gunne AF, Hosman AJ, Cohen DB, et al. A methodological systematic review on surgical site infections following spinal surgery: part 1: risk factors. Spine (Phila Pa 1976). 2012;37(24):2017-33.
11. Kerby JD, Griffin RL, Maclennan P, et al. Stress-induced hyperglycemia, not diabetic hyperglycemia, is associated with higher mortality in trauma. Annals of Surgery. 2012;256(3):446-52.
12. Ahmed AA, Mooar PA, Kleiner M, et al. Hypertensive patients show delayed wound healing following total hip arthroplasty. PLoS One. 2011;6(8):e23224.
13. Fleisher LA, Beckman JA, Brown KA, et al. ACC/AHA 2007 Guidelines on Perioperative Cardiovascular Evaluation and Care for Noncardiac Surgery: Executive Summary: A Report of the American College of Cardiology/American Heart Association Task Force on Practice Guidelines. J Am Coll Cardiol. 2007;50(17):1707-32.
14. Ravi B, Croxford R, Hollands S, et al. Increased risk of complications following total joint arthroplasty in patients with rheumatoid arthritis. Arthritis Rheumatol. 2014;66(2):254-63.
15. Somayaji R, Barnabe C, Martin L. Risk factors for infection following total joint arthroplasty in rheumatoid arthritis. Open Rheumatol J. 2013;7:119-24.

16. Grennan DM, Gray J, Loudon J, et al. Methotrexate and early postoperative complications in patients with rheumatoid arthritis undergoing elective orthopaedic surgery. Ann Rheum Dis. 2001;60(3):214-7.
17. Murata K, Yasuda T, Ito H, et al. Lack of increase in postoperative complications with low-dose methotrexate therapy in patients with rheumatoid arthritis undergoing elective orthopedic surgery. Mod Rheumatol. 2006;16(1):14-9.
18. Carpenter MT, West SG, Vogelgesang SA, et al. Postoperative joint infections in rheumatoid arthritis patients on methotrexate therapy. Orthopedics. 1996;19:207-10.
19. Bridges SL Jr, Lopez-Mendez A, Han KH, et al. Should methotrexate be discontinued before elective orthopedic surgery in patients with rheumatoid arthritis? J Rheumatol 1991;18(7):984-8.
20. Drapeau CM, Pan A, Bellacosa C, et al. Surgical site infections in HIV-infected patients: results from an Italian prospective multicenter observational study. Infection. 2009;37(5):455-60.
21. Madiba TE, Muckart DJ, Thomson SR. Human immunodeficiency disease: how should it affect surgical decision making? World J Surg. 2009;33(5):899-909.
22. George N Guild, Thomas J Moore, Whitney Barnes, et al. CD4 count is associated with postoperative infection in patients with orthopaedic trauma who are HIV positive. Clin Orthop Relat Res. 2012;470(5):1507-12.
23. Howard NE, Phaff M, Aird J, et al. Does human immunodeficiency virus status affect early wound healing in open surgically stabilised tibial fractures?: A prospective study. Bone Joint J. 2013;95-B(12):1703-7.
24. Kigera JW, Straetemans M, Vuhaka SK, et al. Is there an increased risk of post-operative surgical site infection after orthopaedic surgery in HIV patients? A systematic review and meta-analysis. PLoS One. 2012;7(8):e42254.
25. Guild GN, Moore TJ, Barnes W, et al. CD4 count is associated with postoperative infection in patients with orthopaedic trauma who are HIV positive. Clin Orthop Relat Res. 2012;470(5):1507-12.
26. Tomas T. Patient-related risk factors for infected total arthroplasty. Acta Chir Orthop Traumatol Cech. 2008;75(6):451-6.

27. Drancourt M, Argenson JN, Tissot DH, et al. Psoriasis is a risk factor for hip-prosthesis infection. Eur J Epidemiol. 1997;13(2):205-7.
28. Pack-Mabien A, Haynes J Jr. A primary care provider's guide to preventive and acute care management of adults and children with sickle cell disease. J Am Acad Nurse Pract. 2009;21(5):250-7.
29. Ross C. A trauma patient with sickle cell anaemia. J Emerg Nurs. 1997;23(3):211-3.
30. Smetana GW, Conde MV. Preoperative pulmonary update. Clin Geriatr Med. 2008;24(4):607-24.
31. Kaye KS, Sloane R, Sexton DJ, et al. Risk factors for surgical siteinfections in older people. J Am Geriatr Soc. 2006;54(3): 391-6.
32. Koutsoumbelis, Hughes AP, Girardi FP, et al. Risk factors for postoperative infection following posterior lumbar instrumented arthrodesis. J Bone Joint Surg Am. 20117;93(17):1627-33.
33. Bohensky MA, deSteiger R, Kondogiannis C, et al. Adverse outcomes associated with elective knee arthroscopy: a population-based cohort study. Arthroscopy. 2013;29(4):716-25.
34. Miric A, Inacio MC, Namba RS. Can total knee arthroplasty be safely performed in patients with chronic renal disease? Acta Orthop. 2014;85(1):71-8.
35. Chen TH, Matyal R. The management of antiplatelet therapy in patients with coronary stents undergoing non-cardiac surgery. Semin Cardiothorac Vasc Anesth. 2010;14(4):256-73.
36. Grines CL, Bonow RO, Casey DE Jr, et al. Prevention of premature discontinuation of dual antiplatelet therapy in patients with coronary artery stents: a science advisory from the American Heart Association, American College of Cardiology, Society for Cardiovascular Angiography and Interventions, American College of Surgeons, and American Dental Association, with representation from the American College of Physicians. Circulation. 2007;115(6) 813-18.
37. Rossini R, Bramucci E, Castiglioni B, et al. Coronary stenting and surgery: perioperative management of antiplatelet therapy in patients undergoing surgery after coronary stent implantation. G Ital Cardiol (Rome). 2012;13(7-8):528-51.

38. Anderson JL, Adams CD, Antman EM, et al. 2012 ACCF/AHA focused update incorporated into the ACCF/AHA 2007 guidelines for the management of patients with unstable angina/non–ST-elevation myocardial infarction: a report of the American College of Cardiology Foundation/American Heart Association Task Force on Practice Guidelines. Circulation. 2013;127(23):e663-828.
39. Ferraris VA, Saha SP, Oestreich, et al. 2012 update to sts practice guidelines: anti-platelet drugs in cardiac and non-cardiac operations. Ann Thorac Surg. 2012;94(5):1761-81.
40. Hongo RH, Ley J, Dick SE, et al. The effect of clopidogrel in combination with aspirin when given before coronary artery bypasses grafting. J Am Coll Cardiol. 2002;40(2):231-7.
41. Chu MW, Wilson SR, Novick RJ, et al. Does clopidogrel increase blood loss following coronary artery bypass surgery? Ann Thorac Surg. 2004;78(5)1536-41.
42. Blasco-Colmenares E, Trish M Perl, Guallar E, et al. Aspirin plus clopidogrel and risk of infection after coronary artery bypass surgery. Arch Intern Med. 2009;169(8):788-96.
43. Little JW, Jacobson JJ, Lockhart PB, et al. The dental treatment of patients with joint replacements: a position paper from the American Academy of Oral Medicine. J Am Dent Assoc. 2010; 141:667-71.
44. Joseph JJ, Pillai A, Bramley D. Clopidogrel in orthopaedic patients: a review of current practice in Scotland. Thromb J. 2007;5:6.
45. American Dental Association, American Academy of Orthopaedic Surgeons. Advisory statement. Antibiotic prophylaxis for dental patients with total joint replacements. J Am Dent Assoc. 1997;128(7):1004-8.
46. American Dental Association, American Academy of Orthopedic Surgeons. Advisory statement: antibiotic prophylaxis for dental patients with total joint replacements. J Am Dent Assoc. 2003;134(7):895-9.
47. American Academy of Orthopedic Surgeons. Information statement: antibiotic prophylaxis for bacteremia in patients with joint replacements. [online]. Available from www.aaos.org/about/papers/advistmt/1033.asp [Accessed April 13, 2012].

48. Panagiotis Koulouvaris, Peter Sculco, Eileen Finerty, et al. Relationship between perioperative urinary tract infection and deep infection after joint arthroplasty. Clinical Orthopaedics and Related Research. 2009:467(7);1859-67.
49. Ollivere BJ, Ellahee N, Logan K. Asymptomatic urinary tract colonisation predisposes to superficial wound infection in elective orthopaedic surgery. Int Orthop. 2009;33(3):847-850.
50. Bouvet C, Lübbeke A, Bandi C, et al. Is there any benefit in preoperative urinary analysis before elective total joint replacement? Bone Joint J 2014;96-B(3):390-4.
51. Yeshitela B, Gebre-Selassie S, Feleke Y. Asymptomatic bacteriuria and symptomatic urinary tract infections (UTI) in patients with diabetes mellitus in Tikur Anbessa Specialized University Hospital, Addis Ababa, Ethiopia. Ethiop Med J. 2012;50(3):239-49.
52. Thomas Nelius, Stephanie Filleur, Jonathan S Nelson. Asymptomatic bacteriuria: significance for different patient population–InTechOpen, Published on: 2011-09-30.
53. Harris AH, Reeder R, Ellerbe L, et al. Preoperative alcohol screening scores: association with complications in men undergoing total joint arthroplasty. J Bone Joint Surg Am. 2011; 93(4):321-327.
54. Singh JA, Houston TK, Ponce BA, et al. Smoking as a risk factor for short-term outcomes following primary total hip and total knee replacement in veterans. Arthritis Care Res (Hoboken). 2011; 63(10):1365-74.
55. Sørensen LT. Wound healing and infection in surgery. The clinical impact of smoking and smoking cessation: a systematic review and meta-analysis. Arch Surg. 2012;147(4):373-83.
56. Tonnesen H, Nielsen PR, Lauritzen JB, et al. Smoking and alcohol intervention before surgery: evidence for best practice. British Journal of Anaesthesia. 2009;102(3):297-306.
57. Wu C, Qu X, Liu F, Li H, et al. Risk factors for peri-prosthetic joint infection after total hip arthroplasty and total knee arthroplasty in Chinese patient. PLoS One. 2014;9(4):e95300.
58. Eoin Sheehan, Javad Parvizi. Blood transfusions can increase the risk of infection in orthopaedic patients. Orthopaedics Today, January 2010.

59. Ran Schwarzkopf, Christine Chung, BA, Justin J. Park, et al. Effects of perioperative blood product use on surgical site infection following thoracic and lumbar spinal surgery. Spine (Phila Pa 1976). 2010;35(3):340-36.
60. Nicholson JA, Dowrick AS, Liew SM. Nutritional status and short-term outcome of hip arthroplasty. J Orthop Surg (Hong Kong). 2012;20(3):331-5.
61. Brian G Webb, David M Lichtman, Russell A Wagner. Risk factors in total joint arthroplasty: comparison of infection rates in patients with different socioeconomic backgrounds. Orthopaedics. 2008;31(5):445.
62. Jennifer Warner. Obese Patients Have a Higher Risk of Complications Following Surgery. WebMD Health News. March 14, 2007.
63. Obese Patients Face Increased Risks for Infection and Dislocation Following Revision Hip Replacement Surgery. Arthritis Care Research News Alerts. 2008;59(4):738-745.
64. Jämsen E, Nevalainen P, Eskelinen A, et al. Obesity, diabetes, and preoperative hyperglycemia as predictors of periprosthetic joint infection: a single-center analysis of 7181 primary hip and knee replacements for osteoarthritis. J Bone Joint Surg Am. 2012;94(14):e101.
65. Krushell RJ, Fingeroth RJ. Primary total knee arthroplasty in morbidly obese patients: a 5- to 14-year follow-up study. J Arthroplasty. 2007; 22(6 suppl 2):77-80.
66. Dowsey MM, Choong PF. Obese diabetic patients are at substantial risk for deep infection after primary TKA. Clin Orthop Relat Res. 2009;467(6)1577-81.
67. Malinzak RA, Ritter MA, Berend ME, et al. Morbidly obese, diabetic, younger, and unilateral joint arthroplasty patients have elevated total joint arthroplasty infection rates. J Arthroplasty. 2009;24(6 suppl):84-7.
68. Samson AJ, Mercer GE, Campbell DG. Total knee replacement in the morbidly obese: a literature review. ANZ Journal of Surgery. 2010;80(9):595-9.
69. Bozic KJ, Ward DT, Lau EC, et al. Risk factors for periprosthetic joint infection following primary total hip arthroplasty: a case control study. J Arthroplasty. 2014;29(1):154-6.

70. Kaye KS, Schmader KE, Sawyer R. Surgical site infection in the elderly population. Clin Infect Dis. 2004;39(12):1835-41.
71. Lee J, Singletary R, Schmader K, et al. Surgical site infection in the elderly following orthopaedic surgery. Risk factors and outcomes. J Bone Joint Surg Am. 2006;88(8):1705-12.
72. Kaye K, Caughlan K, Sloane RJ, et al. Risk factors for surgical site infections (SSI) in the elderly: a multi-centre study. American Geriatrics Society Annual Meeting (Las Vegas). 20 May. 2004.
73. Skråmm I, Fossum Moen AE, Arøen A, et al. Surgical Site Infections in Orthopaedic Surgery Demonstrate Clones Similar to Those in Orthopaedic Staphylococcus aureus Nasal Carriers. J Bone Joint Surg Am. 2014;96(11):882-8.
74. Perl TM. Prevention of Staphylococcus aureus infections among surgical patients: beyond traditional perioperative prophylaxis. Surgery. 2003;134(5 Suppl):S10-7.
75. Malviya S, Voepel-Lewis T, Siewert M, et al. Risk factors for adverse postoperative outcomes in children presenting for cardiac surgery with upper respiratory tract infections. Anesthesiology. 2003;98(3):628-32.
76. Elwood T, Bailey K. The pediatric patient and upper respiratory infections. Best Pract Res Clin Anaesthesiol. 2005;19(1):35-46.
77. Tait, Alan R Malviya, Shobha. Anesthesia for the child with an upper respiratory tract infection: still a dilemma? Anesthesia and Analgesia. 2005;100(1):59-65.

Patient and Operative Site Preparation

Madhav Borate, Hemant M Wakankar

INTRODUCTION

Endogenous microbial flora (particularly *Staphylococcus aureus* and *Streptococcus* species) are the most common source of surgical site infection (SSI). The term SSI is more appropriate than 'surgical wound contaminant' because it includes infection that directly results from surgical procedures that involve other areas of the body as well, such as organs or internal spaces that are manipulated during the operation.

Surgical site infections are classified by the Centers for Disease Control and Prevention (CDC) as incisional (infection of the actual site of the surgical incision) or organ/space (infection of an anatomic part that was manipulated during the operation). Incisional SSIs are further classified as superficial (involving the skin and subcutaneous tissue) or deep (involving deep soft tissue layers such as incisional fascia and muscle). To be considered an SSI, an infection must occur within 30 days of the surgical procedure. This chapter deals with patients and operative site preparations, so as to minimize the SSIs.

HAIR REMOVAL/CLIPPING

Is hair removal or clipping necessary? What is the proper method of hair removal prior to surgery?

We recommend clipping or depilator as a preferred method for hair removal, only if it comes in the area of incision and surgical field. Hair removal creams can also be used as an alternative. Shaving is not advisable for hair removal.

Explanation

Removal of hair from the surgical site is necessary, only if it comes in the surgical field. Having hairless surgical site may assist the suturing, application of dressings and reduce potential infection. Clipping or epilators are best methods for hair removal. Shaving is not the preferred mode for hair removal as it causes abrasions during the process and cause bacterial growth. A recent systematic review of randomized controlled trials (RCT) conclusively stated that the hair removal by clipping had a lower rate of SSI as compared to shaving.[1] Many other studies have also shown hair clipping to be superior to shaving.[2-4] Some institutes use depilatory creams as a method of hair removal.

What is the appropriate time and place for hair removal?

Hair removal, whenever necessary, should be done as close to the surgery time as possible. Hair removal can be done in the patient's room or a recovery room.

Explanation

Hair removal should be performed as close to the time of the surgical procedure as possible. One study that was conducted to determine the appropriate time of hair removal showed that clipping done on the morning of the surgery had lower rates of SSI.[5] Another observation that studied the effect of shaving versus depilatory creams on SSI showed that shaving done just before surgery had lower incidence of SSI as compared to shaving done 24 hours before surgery.[6]

The CDC recommends hair removal preoperatively, only if it interferes with the incision site. If the hair removal is necessary, it is performed immediately prior to the surgery preferably with clippers.[7]

As there is lack of research as to where the hair removal should be performed, we recommend that it should be performed in the recovery room or the ward just before shifting the patient to operation theater (OT). It should be done by trained surgical team or nursing staff.

How should the surgical site be prepared?

The surgical site should be prepared by scrubbing with 7.5% povidone–iodine (PI) for minimum 3 minutes with final cleaning by isopropyl alcohol. Surgical site can also be prepared by chlorhexidine gluconate with 70% isopropyl alcohol as combined solution where second step is not needed. It is important to wait for about 20 seconds and let the alcohol dry on the skin after its application.

Explanation

Iodine/iodophors act by oxidation of the cell wall membrane and have minimal residual action. Iodine acts by decreasing the oxygen requirements of aerobic microorganisms. Iodine interferes at the level of the respiratory chain of the microorganisms by blocking the transport of electrons through electrophilic reactions with the enzymes of the respiratory chain.[8,9] Alcohol causes denaturation of proteins and has a rapid mechanism of action. Hence, the combination of alcohol and iodophors provides very good antisepsis.[10] Isopropyl alcohol is more potent against bacteria, while ethyl alcohol is more potent against viruses. Alcohols do not have sporicidal activity. The antimicrobial activity of alcohols is optimal in concentrations between 60 and 90%. It should be allowed to dry on the skin.[11,12] Iodine, however, has shown to cause allergic reactions in some patients. Hence, a skin testing is recommended prior to the usage of iodine scrub.

Chlorhexidine has been considered to be one of the best antiseptic solutions. Chlorhexidine was claimed by Harold et al.[13] to be an inhibitor of both membrane-bound and soluble ATPase as well as of net K⁺ uptake. It has a biphasic effect on protoplast lysis, with reduced lyses at higher biguanide concentrations. The uptake by bacteria[14] and yeasts[15] was shown to be extremely rapid, with a maximum effect occurring within 20 seconds. One of the studies conducted with a small sample of people showed decreased microbial colonization with a chlorhexidine wash given over a 5 day period.[16] Another meta-analysis showed that alcoholic chlorhexidine had better efficacy than alcoholic PI. A two-step intervention using PI scrub and paint followed by alcohol showed significantly better efficacy over PI.[17] However, care should be taken to avoid excess use of chlorhexidine as excess use shows no benefit and may cause skin irritation.[18,19]

What should be the draping material used during surgery?

We advise the use disposable impervious drapes with a sterile plastic sheet (8–10 μ) underneath the drape. In case cost is a constraint, the use of reusable drapes (linen) with the final draping done with the help of a disposable drape is advised.

Explanation

Reusable drapes are linen drapes that are permeable to liquids. Woven and non-woven materials vary in their ability to resist bacterial strikethrough. Drape materials may demonstrate different levels of permeability depending upon the penetrating particle (aqueous fluid, albumin or bacteria).[20-22] While passage of the bacteria through dry drape does happen, the strike-through rate of bacteria is enhanced when the drape is wet because of normal saline or blood and diminished when wetted by antiseptic solutions.[23]

Fabrics having smaller pore size are considered to have better barrier efficacy. As a principle, the pore size of the fabric must be smaller than the size of microorganism or its carrier. The mean pore width of a reusable drape is 120.4 ± 26.33 μ.

There is a significant increase in pore size as observed at 1st laundering to 5th laundering, 10th laundering to 15th laundering and at 15th laundering to 20th laundering respectively.[24,25,26] It is due to the reason that repeated laundering increases the pore size of the fabric. The laundering procedure and the detergent/soap being used for laundering surgical gown are also damaging the fabric. Sterilization is also one of the damaging causes. Steam helps the pores to grow large. The porosity of the fabrics increased after laundering, which indicates that the fabric had a more open structure, and that microorganisms and liquids could pass through the fabric structure more easily.[25,26]

Disposable woven drapes are superior to reusable cotton/linen drapes in resisting bacterial penetration. When wetted by normal saline, reusable woven drapes were penetrated by bacteria within 30 minutes, while the majority of disposable woven drapes were not.[27,28] A sterile plastic sheet can be used underneath the drape, which has a pore width of 8–10 μ as an additional protection to prevent leaking of fluids in case of tearing of the disposable drape.

For better maintenance of sterilization, we advise the use of impermeable disposable surgical drapes. This will prevent leaking of fluids. This will also maintain adequate sterilization.

Is there any difference in preparing patient with skin lesions?

Active skin lesions, if present in the vicinity of the surgical site should be treated first prior to surgery. Elective surgical procedures should not be performed in case of active lesions. Incision should not be placed over an active lesion. In case of lesions like psoriasis or eczema, the surgery should be delayed and that performed only after optimization of the patient.

Explanation

Elective surgery should be delayed in cases where patients have active lesions in the vicinity of the surgical site.

Ulcerations, causing the break in continuity of the skin, have a high risk of infection. A prospective study concluded that there was significant rise of the SSI in patients with active ulceration of the skin.[29]

There are no studies evaluating the risk of SSIs when incisions are placed through the eczematous or psoriatic skin lesions. Two studies have reported high rate of SSIs in patients diagnosed with psoriasis or eczema.[30,31] However, the study did not evaluate whether the high rates of infection was due to the skin lesions or due to the generalized immunosuppression. It was shown that there were increased bacterial load on the psoriatic skin.[32] Hence placing incisions over the psoriatic or eczematous skin should be avoided. Elective surgery should be delayed and should be performed only after optimization of the patient.

When should the change of clothes to clean OT clothes be made in a patient posted for surgery?

Change of clothes to clean OT clothes should be made as close as possible to the surgery time. Probably just before leaving the ward room to go to the OT recovery or right there in the OT recovery should be done.

Explanation

There is no study that clearly states as to where the change of clothes to clean clothes be made. We recommend change of clothes from the patient clothes to clean OT clothes should be made as close as possible to the operating room, which will decrease the bacterial transmission of bacteria as the patient is being shifted from the room to the operation theater. There is no need to provide autoclaved clothes to the patients, however, evidence for or against this practice is not available.

In case of elective surgery, the patient should be advised to take bath with an antiseptic soap in the night prior to surgery and then again in the morning of the surgery and then the clothes should be changed.

In case of non-union surgery or in previously casted limb, the limb should be given a 7.5% PI scrub bath (with prior skin testing) or with a chlorhexidine gluconate solution after hair removal and then the clothes should be changed.

Is operative site preparation different in compound fractures?

Diluted iodine-based agents with normal saline are preferred in cases of compound injuries. A 0.02% chlorhexidine solution is also preferred for wound irrigation. Alcohol-based antiseptics are not to be used on open wounds.

Explanation

An ideal antiseptic for use in open wounds should possess effective bactericidal action and be nontoxic to tissues and not interfere with or delay healing.[33]

Iodine-based surgical antiseptics are effective against a wide range of gram positive and negative organisms including methicillin-resistant *Staphylococcus aureus* (MRSA), as well as tubercle bacillus, fungi and viruses. Their mechanism of action is via oxidation after penetration of the cell wall. Iodophors such as PI are iodine formulations prepared with a stabilizing agent that liberates free iodine and can be prepared in aqueous or alcohol preparations. Commercially prepared PI solutions or paints contain approximately 90% water, 8.5% PI and 1% iodine. PI scrubs contain 7.5% PI, 0.75% available iodine and detergent. PI may be inactivated by blood or serum proteins, but as long as they are present on the skin exert a bacteriostatic effect. PI has not been found to promote or inhibit wound healing.[34] Systemic absorption of iodine can occur and in rare cases has led to iodine toxicosis and death; care should thus be taken when using this preparation especially in high-risk populations such as severe burn victims and newborns.[34]

Chlorhexidine was also found to be relatively safe for use as a surgical wound irrigation solution. Only the higher concentrations (0.05%) caused slight tissue toxicity in rats. Lower concentrations (0.02%) are recommended for wound irrigation.[34]

The use of 3% hydrogen peroxide helps in removing the foreign material that causes contamination. A wash should be given with normal saline. Hydrogen peroxide appears not to negatively influence wound healing, but it is also ineffective in reducing the bacterial count.[34] However, it may be useful as a chemical debriding agent. The American Medical Association concluded that the effervescence of hydrogen peroxide might provide some mechanical benefit in loosening debris and necrotic tissue of the wound.[34] Alcohol-based antiseptics should not be used on open wounds as they cause damage to the soft tissues by their action of protein denaturation.

SUMMARY

1. Hair removal is necessary only when it comes in the area of incision or surgical field. Hair removal should be done as close to surgery time as possible, preferably in the wards just before shifting to OT. Clipping or depilator is the best method to remove hair. Shaving is not recommended.
2. The surgical site should be prepared by scrubbing with 7.5% povidone–iodine for minimum 3 minutes with final cleaning by isopropyl alcohol.
3. For draping use of disposable impervious drapes with a sterile plastic sheet (8–10 microns) underneath the drape is recommended. In case cost is a constraint, the use of reusable drapes (linen) with the final draping done using a disposable drape is advised.
4. For compound fractures iodine-based solutions are recommended. Alcohol-based solutions are not recommended for compound fractures.

REFERENCES

1. Tanner J, Norrie P, Melen K. Preoperative hair removal to reduce surgical site infection. Cochrane Database Syst Rev. 2011(11):CD004122.
2. Balthazar ER, Colt JD, Nichols RL. Preoperative hair removal: a random prospective study of shaving versus clipping. South Med J. 1982;75(7):799-801.
3. Ko W, Lazenby WD, Zelano JA, et al. Effects of shaving methods and intra-operative irrigation on suppurative mediastinitis after bypass operations. Ann Thorac Surg. 1992;53(2):301-5.
4. Sellick JA Jr, Stelmach M, Mylotte JM. Surveillance of surgical wound infections following open heart surgery. Infect Control Hosp Epidemiol. 1991;12(10):591-6.
5. Alexander JW, Fischer JE, Boyajian M, et al. The influence of hair-removal methods on wound infections. Arch Surg. 1983;118(3):347-52.
6. Seropian R, Reynolds BM. Wound infections after preoperative depilatory versus razor preparation. Am J Surg. 1971;121(3):251-4.
7. Reichman DE, Greenberg JA. Reducing surgical site infections: a review. Rev Obstet Gynecol. 2009 Fall;2(4): 212–21.
8. Dauphin A and Darbord JC. Hygiène hospitalière pratique, 2nd edition. Association de pharmacie hospitalière de l'Ile-de-France. Editions médicales internationales, 1988. p. 715.
9. Russell AD. Principles of antimicrobial activity. In: Block SS (Ed). Disinfection, sterilization and preservation, 3rd edition. Philadelphia: Lea and Febiger; 1983. pp. 717-45.
10. Cheng CK, Mart JP, Robertson H, et al. Quantitative analysis of bacteria in forefoot surgery: a comparision of skin preparation techniques. J Bone Joint Surg Br. 2011; 64(4):93.
11. Gerald McDonnell, A. Denver Russell. Antiseptics and disinfectants: activity, action, and resistance. ClinMicrobiol Rev. 1999;12(1):147-79.
12. Klein M, Deforest A. Principles of viral inactivation. In: Block SS (Ed). Disinfection, sterilization and preservation, 3rd edition. Philadelphia: Lea and Febiger; 1983. pp. 422-34.

13. Harold FM, Baarda JR, Baron C, et al. Dio and chlorhexidine. Inhibition of membrane bound ATPase and of cation transport in *Streptococcus faecalis*. Biochim Biophys Acta. 1969;183: 129-36.
14. Fitzgerald KA, Davies A, Russell AD. Uptake of 14C-chlorhexidine diacetate to *Escherichia coli* and *Pseudomonas aeruginosa* and its release by azolectin. FEMS MicrobiolLett. 1989;60:327-32.
15. Hiom SJ, Furr JR, Russell AD, et al. Effects of chlorhexidine diacetate on Candida albicans, C. glabrata and Saccharomyces cerevisiae. J ApplBacteriol. 1992;72:335-40.
16. Parienti JJ, Thibon P, Heller R, et al. Antisepsie Chirurgicale des mains Study Group. Hand-rubbing with an aqueous alcoholic solution vs traditional surgicalhand-scrubbing and 30-day surgical site infection rates: a randomized equivalencestudy. JAMA. 2002;288(6):722-7.
17. Yammine K, Harvey A, Efficacy of preparation solutions and cleansing techniques on contamination of the skin in foot and ankle surgery. A systematic review and meta-analysis. Bone Joint J. 2013;95-B(4):498-503.
18. Lilly HA, Lowbury EJ, Wilkins MD. Limits to progressive reduction of resident skin bacteria by disinfection. J ClinPathol. 1979;32(4):382-5.
19. Lowbury EJ, Lilly HA. Use of 4 per cent chlorhexidine detergent solution (Hibiscrub) and other methods of skin disinfection. Br Med J. 1973;1(5852):510-5.
20. Blom A, Estela C, Bowker K, et al. The passage of bacteria through surgical drapes. Ann R CollSurg Engl. 2000;82(6):405-7.
21. Ha'eri GB, Wiley AM. Wound contamination through drapes and gowns: a study using tracer particles. Clin Orthop Relat Res. 1981;(154):181-4.
22. Mackintosh CA, Lidwell OM. The evaluation of fabrics in relation to their use as protective garments in nursing and surgery. III. Wet penetration and contact transfer of particles through clothing. J Hyg (Lond). 1980;85(3):393-403.
23. Blom AW, Gozzard C, Heal J, et al. Bacterial strike-through of re-usable surgical drapes: the effect of different wetting agents. J Hosp Infect. 2002;52(1):52-5.

24. Kishwar F, Hanif A, Kalsoom S, et al. Comparison of Pore Size Analysis of Existing and Experimental Surgical Gowns. Professional Med J. 2014;21(4):804-9.
25. AST (2012). Recommended Standards of Practice for Surgical Drapes. Retrieved from Standards_of_Practice/RSOP_Surgical_Drapes.pdf.
26. Leonas KK and Jinkins RS. The relationship of selected fabric characteristics and the barrier effectiveness of surgical gown fabric. Am J Infect Control. 1997;16-23.
27. Blom AW, Barnett A, Ajitsaria P, et al. Resistance of disposable drapes to bacterial penetration. J Orthop Surg (Hong Kong). 2007;15(3):267-9.
28. Johnston DH, Fairclough JA, Brown EM, et al. Rate of bacterial re-colonization of the skin after preparation: four methods compared. Br J Surg. 1987;74(1):64.
29. Penington A. Ulceration and antihypertensive use are risk factors for infection after skin lesion excision. ANZ J Surg. 2010;80(9):642-5.
30. Menon TJ, Wroblewski BM. Charnley low-friction arthroplasty in patients with psoriasis. Clin Orthop Relat Res. 1983;(176):127-8.
31. Stern SH, Insall JN, Windsor RE, et al. Total knee arthroplasty in patients with psoriasis. Clin Orthop Relat Res. 1989;(248):108-10;discussion 111.
32. Aly R, Maibach HE, Mandel A. Bacterial flora in psoriasis. Br J Dermatol. 1976;95(6):603-6.
33. WL Estes Jr. The use of antiseptics in the treatment of open wounds. The American Journal of Surgery. 1940;47(2):369-74.
34. Drosou A, Falabella A, Kirsner RS. Antiseptics on Wounds: An Area of Controversy. Wounds. 2003;15(5):799-801.

8

Intraoperative Protocols

Amol Narkhede, Anil Jain, Parag K Sancheti, Hemant M Wakankar

INTRODUCTION

In this chapter we will discuss the issues related to intraoperative surgical practices to reduce the incidence of surgical site infection (SSI). Some of the important issues are management of infected cases, effect of prolonged duration of surgery on rate of infection, role of incise draping in reducing SSI, necessity of change of knife blade during surgery for deeper dissection, when to change suction tips, any difference in incidence of SSI with use of staples and suture materials, perioperative patient warming, etc. We will discuss all these points.

Does the prolonged surgery (> 2 hours) time have any effect on incidence of infection?

Yes. Prolonged surgery time (> 2 hours) is associated with increased risk of infection and all attempts to minimize the surgical time should be done. Namba et al reported 9% increase in the risk of deep SSI per 15 minutes increment increase in operative time. In case, the surgical time extends more than 2 hours then frequent wound wash/lavage should be given with normal saline.

Explanation

In study by Peersman et al, 113 infected patients were matched with 236 controls and nominal variables were statistically processed. Patients without infections (n = 236) had surgery durations of 94 ± 28 min and patients with infection (n = 104) had durations of 127 ± 45 min (p < 0.001). The results confirm that the duration of the surgical procedure can be used as a risk predictor for SSI in total knee replacement (TKR).[1] Operative time approaching 3 hours and open fractures are related to an increased overall risk for SSI after open plating of the tibial plateau. Dual incision approaches with bicolumnar plating do not appear to expose the patient to increased risk compared to single incision approaches.[2] The risk of SSI varied according to the length of surgery with the greatest risk for procedures, which lasted 120 minutes or more.[3] Preoperative and intraoperative risk factors for SSIs are—inappropriate use of antimicrobial prophylaxis, infection at remote site not treated prior to surgery, shaving the site vs clipping, long duration of surgery, improper skin preparation, improper surgical team hand preparation, environment of the operating room (ventilation, sterilization), surgical attire and drapes asepsis.[4-6]

Many studies have shown increased duration of surgery, which is associated with increased risk of infection. But some difficult surgeries like polytrauma, complex fractures; those associated with vascular injury, nonunions and revision joint replacements surgeries are inherently associated with prolong surgery time. These cases should be approached in a systematic manner. Entire OT staff should be educated regarding the importance of decreasing the surgery time and techniques required to do so without compromising the quality of work. Surgical steps should be planned, skilled staff should be available for such kind of cases so that complications are avoided or reduced, which in turn will result in reduction of surgery time. An additional antibiotic dose or single dose of broad-spectrum antibiotic should be considered when surgery time is prolonged excessively or more than half-life of the antibiotic dose used at the beginning of the procedure.

What is the role of incise draping in orthopedic surgeries? Should the incise draping be impregnated with antimicrobials or clear incise drapes should be used?

Incised drapes are used to decrease the incidence of SSIs. Clear drapes restrict the movements of skin flora during surgical procedure, while impregnated drapes provide sustained antimicrobial activity during surgery. Thus, it seems an impregnated incised drape would be more suitable for the same.

Explanation

Antimicrobial incised drapes effectively reduces the levels of microorganisms associated with post-operative infection.[7] Iodine impregnated incise drapes reduce the likelihood of skin recolonization after prepping, and thus reduce the risk of wound contamination by skin flora, which is a common cause of SSI. A non-impregnated incise drape does not have the iodophor active agent, but simply immobilizes the skin flora as it continues to grow throughout the procedure. All Ioban antimicrobial incise drapes offer the following:

- Iodophor for sustained antimicrobial activity throughout the procedure
- A conformable film that adheres to body contours
- Breathable ensuring adhesion to the skin.

Iodine impregnated incise drapes are supported by clinical evidence covering a variety of surgical procedures and should be used following preoperative skin antisepsis.[8]

The uses of plastic adhesive incise drapes to prevent contamination of the wound from skin infections has been used for at least 50 years. Reports of controlled studies have mixed results, some showing some benefit whereas, others report no benefit. A major part of these discrepancies is related to differences in the composition of the drapes themselves. The drapes available after 1985 are more pliable, have increased water vapor transmission and a more aggressive adhesive, which has an iodophor incorporated. Use of the older drapes without the iodophor has been associated with an increase in separation of the drape from the skin edges at the incision.

One study showed that if lifting at the edge of the skin occurs, the infection rate was six-fold greater when compared to operations in which the incise drape did not lift. The studies before use of the new drape, in general, showed no benefit or an increase in infections when compared to no drape at all. Even when there was no difference in postoperative wound infection rates, the number of viable organisms on the surface of the skin at the completion of the operation was decreased by the use of the iodophor-containing drapes. A variant of this concept, application of a cyanoacrylate based 'microbial sealant' to the operative site to trap microbes on the skin has recently been introduced. This product has been shown to reduce wound colonization, but its ability to reduce infection needs further study before general recommendation.[9,10]

Should the knife blade be changed after skin incision for deeper dissection?

Knife blade should not be changed after skin incision for deeper dissection.

Explanation

It is a common practice among surgeons of all specialties to discard the scalpel blade used for the skin incision and to use a fresh blade for deeper dissection. The logic being although the skin surface is rendered sterile by preoperative scrubbing, as much as 20% of skin bacteria may remain in skin's sweat glands and hair follicles and are potentially the source of wound flora. Another school of thought believes that the knife is blunted after cutting the skin. However, evidence suggests the practice of changing the blade is unnecessary.

Investigators cultured skin and deep dissection blades in orthopedic surgeries and reported no correlations among contaminated skin blades, deep blades and wound infections. A prospective, randomized study of 586 patients showed no difference in wound infection rates between one and two blade surgeries and only one positive blade culture.

It is not clear if these data can be extended to contaminated orthopedic cases such as open fractures. The economic impact of discarding a scalpel blade is minor compared with other surgical costs. Nonetheless, it is a good example of a common practice that continues despite evidence pointing to the contrary.[11]

The scalpel blades used during 187 operations were cultured. At each procedure the knife used to incise the skin was discarded immediately and a fresh knife was used to complete the operation. The results showed that there was no difference in the bacterial growth between the two knives. From these results it would appear that the practice of changing blades after incising the skin is an unnecessary precaution in the prevention of bacterial contamination of clean wounds.[12-14]

How often should the suction tips be changed during surgery? Which type of suction tips should be used whether metallic or disposable?

Suction tips should be changed every 60 minutes during surgery to reduce the incidence of SSIs. Disposable suction tips are always preferred to non-disposable metallic ones.

Explanation

We believe that despite the low risk of deep wound infection, changing the suction tip every hour in long orthopedic procedures or using the on/off switch is well justified in an effort to minimize the chances of deep wound infection.[15,16]

Our recommendation is that suction tips should be changed every 60 minutes during surgery to reduce the incidence of SSIs. The studies have showed increased rates of contamination if suction tips are not changed or changed after long time. Suction tip should enter intramedullary canal of long bones for the time necessary to evacuate the fluid. It should not be left in the canal as it can circulate large amount of ambient air and particles, which can contaminate the surgery.

For metallic suction tips are used autoclave should be used for sterilization for effective cleaning. There are different biological, chemical and mechanical markers to monitor efficacy of autoclave as per Centers for Disease Control and Prevention (CDC) guidelines. For removing particulate matter from suction tips air guns, pressure guns, cleaning brushes, enzymatic cleaning agents/detergents, and ultrasonic cleaning methods are used.

Is there any difference between staples and suture material in reducing the incidence of SSI?

There is no difference between staples and suture material in reducing the incidence of SSI however, staples by virtue of reducing the surgery time may contribute to reduced SSI (specially in prolonged surgeries).

Explanation

After orthopedic surgery, there is a significantly higher risk of developing a wound infection when the wound is closed with staples rather than sutures. This risk is specifically greater in patients who undergo hip surgery. The use of staples for closing hip or knee surgery wounds after orthopedic procedures cannot be recommended, though the evidence comes from studies with substantial methodological limitations. Though we advise orthopedic surgeons to reconsider their use of staples for wound closure, definitive randomized trials are still needed to assess this research question.[17]

A study titled 'blinded prospective randomized controlled trial comparing 2-octyl cyanoacrylate (OCA), subcuticular suture (monocryl) and skin staples for skin closure following total hip and total knee arthroplasty' included 102 hip replacements and 85 of the knee. OCA was associated with less wound discharge in the first 24 hours for both the hip and the knee. However, with total knee replacement there was a trend for a more prolonged wound discharge with OCA. With total hip replacement there was no significant difference between the groups for either early or late complications. Closure of the wound with skin staples was significantly faster than with OCA or suture. There was no significant difference in the length of stay in hospital. Hollander wound evaluation score (cosmesis) or patient satisfaction between the groups at 6 weeks for either hips or knees. This study concludes that skin staples are the skin closure of choice for both hip and knee replacements.[18] One study suggests that 42% of patients report a wound complication with no difference between sutures and staples. It was demonstrated that suturing skin requires more time and staples are more painful to remove.[19]

In another study, there was no difference in healing in all four groups, but staples were easier and faster and had less microorganisms growth around them. Staples are more expensive and more painful on removal when compared to other groups. The main advantage of vicryl rapid was that there was no need for removal and had comparable results. Silk had the same results as the other groups, but is considerably cheaper when compared to the other materials.[20,21]

We recommend that staples should be used for joint replacement surgeries. For long wounds staples reduce closure time. For other surgeries it mainly depends on surgeon's preference and patient's affordability. Although using staples reduces wound closure time facilities for removing staples may not be available at remote places, which is another factor determining whether to use staples or suture material.

What is the role of antibiotics in irrigation solutions during surgery?

Irrigation with normal saline is optimal and adding an antibiotic to irrigation solution has no additional benefit.

> **Explanation**

It is a common practice to add antibiotics to irrigation solutions especially in arthroplasty or open fractures. The logic is to reduce the infection rate especially by gram-positive bacteria, however, quantity and effectiveness of this practice is not yet established. In vivo studies have shown that antibiotics in irrigation solution are not more effective than saline in removing bacteria from bone or steel implants.[22] Antibiotic irrigation has been effective in experimental studies in some types of animal wounds, but human clinical data are unconvincing due to poor study design.[23] A review article published in 1991 by Dirschl and Wilson[24] did support use of triple antibiotic solution (neomycin, polymyxin and bacitracin) and suggested a contact period of one minute for the solution to act. However, they did warn about toxicity and adverse reactions and also development of antibiotic resistance. Anglen in his randomized trial noted that infection rates are similar when using antibiotic irrigation compared to soap water irrigation in open fractures, however, antibiotic irrigation group had more bone healing problems.[25] Thus, the evidence supporting use of antibiotic irrigation solution is not really convincing and we believe saline solutions are the best irrigation solution currently.[11] Also it is the frequency and volume of irrigation and not the bactericidal quality that is more important than bactericidal properties.

Should the infected and contaminated cases be scheduled only after completion of clean cases?

Yes. Infected and contaminated cases should be scheduled only after completion of clean cases.

Explanation

There are many studies that are in favor of infected and contaminated cases being scheduled only after completion of clean cases. Microbiological studies demonstrate long survivorship of common nosocomial pathogens on inanimate surfaces, which theoretically is in support of risk of cross-contamination if adequate care is not taken to disinfect the OT when clean cases are taken after contaminated cases.

Lists should be compiled in a logical format, e.g., infected cases last on the list, latex allergy patients first on the list,[26] whenever possible, infected cases should be placed at the end of the operating list. In some hospitals, a special designated theater may be used.[27] A separate theater should be kept for arthroplasty and arthroscopy case whenever possible. The OT staff should be educated about the importance of personal hygiene and need of strict disinfection practices after contaminated cases. Whenever possible the staffs who have been involved in the contaminated case should not go to next clean case.

SUMMARY

1. Infected and contaminated cases should be scheduled only after completion of clean cases.
2. Prolonged surgery time (> 2 hours) is associated with increased risk of infection.
3. Incised drapes are used to decrease the incidence of SSIs. Clear drapes restrict the movements of skin flora during surgical procedure, while impregnated drapes provide sustained antimicrobial activity during surgery.
4. Knife blade should not be changed after skin incision for deeper dissection.

5. Suction tips should be changed every 60 minutes during surgery to reduce the incidence of SSIs. Disposable suction tips are always preferred to non-disposable metallic ones.
6. There is no difference between staples and suture material in reducing the incidence of SSIs.

REFERENCES

1. Peersman G, Laskin R, Davis J, et al. Prolonged operative time correlates with increased infection rate after total knee arthroplasty. HSS J. 2006;2(1):70-2.
2. Colman M, Wright A, Gruen G, et al. Prolonged operative time increases infection rate in tibial plateau fractures. Injury. 2013;44(2):249-52.
3. Ridgeway S, Wilson J, Charlet A, et al. Infection of the surgical site after arthroplasty of the hip. J Bone Joint Surg Br. 2005;87(6):844-50.
4. Harrop JS, Styliaras JC, Ooi YC, et al. Contributing factors to surgical site infections. J Am Acad Orthop Surg. 2012;20(2):94-101.
5. Greene LR. Guide to the elimination of orthopedic surgery surgical site infections: an executive summary of the Association for Professionals in Infection Control and Epidemiology elimination guide. Am J Infect Control. 2012;40(4):384-6.
6. Parvizi J, Gehrke T. Proceedings of the International consensus meeting on periprosthetic joint infection. Bone joint J. 2013;89.
7. Kramer A, Assadian O, Lademann J. Prevention of postoperative wound infections by covering the surgical field with iodine-impregnated incision drape (Ioban 2). GMS Krankenhhyg Interdiszip. 2010;5(2).
8. Kapadia BH, Pivec R, Johnson AJ, Issa K, et al. Infection prevention methodologies for lower extremity total joint arthroplasty. Expert Rev Med Devices. 2013;10(2):215-24.
9. Alexander JW, Solomkin JS, Edwards MJ. Updated recommendations for control of surgical site infections. Ann Surg. 2011;253(6):1082-93.
10. Parvizi J, Gehrke T. Proceedings of the International consensus meeting on periprosthetic joint infection. Bone joint J. 2013;98.

11. Nirmal C, Tejwani, Igor Immerman. Myths and legends in orthopaedic practice: are we all guilty? Clin Orthop Relat Res. 2008;466(11):2861-72.
12. Fairclough JA, Mackie IG, Mintowt-Czyz W, et al. The contaminated skin-knife. A surgical myth. J Bone Joint Surg Br. 1983;65(2):210.
13. Hill R, Blair S, Neely J, et al. Changing knives a wasteful and unnecessary ritual. Ann R Coll Surg Engl. 1985;67(3):149-51.
14. Parvizi J, Gehrke T. Proceedings of the International consensus meeting on periprosthetic joint infection. Bone joint J. 2013;96.
15. Givissis P, Karataglis D, Antonarakos P, et al. Suction during orthopaedic surgery. How safe is the suction tip? Acta Orthop Belg. 2008;74(4):531-3.
16. Parvizi J, Gehrke T. Proceedings of the International consensus meeting on periprosthetic joint infection. Bone joint J. 2013;97.
17. Smith TO, Sexton D, Mann C, et al. Sutures versus staples for skin closure in orthopaedic surgery: meta-analysis BMJ. 2010;340:c1199.
18. Khan RJ, Fick D, Yao F, et al. A comparison of three methods of wound closure following arthroplasty: a prospective, randomised, controlled trial. J Bone Joint Surg Br. 2006;88(2):238-42.
19. Slade Shantz JA, Vernon J, Morshed S, et al. Sutures versus staples for wound closure in orthopaedic surgery: a pilot randomized controlled trial. Patient Saf Surg. 2013;7(1):6.
20. Muhammad Israr, leo Fa Stassen. The comparison of scalp closure with staples, silk, prolene, vicryl following a Gille's temporal approach for malar/zygomatic complex fracture; a prospective study. Pakistan Oral & Dental Journal. 2013;33 (1): 3-7.
21. Parvizi J, Gehrke T. Proceedings of the International consensus meeting on periprosthetic joint infection. Bone joint J. 2013;107.
22. Anglen J, Apostoles PS, Christensen G, et al. Removal of surface bacteria by irrigation. J Orthop Res. 1996;14(2):251-4.
23. Anglen JO. Wound irrigation in musculoskeletal injury. J Am Acad Orthop Surg. 2001;9(4):219-26.

24. Dirschl DR, Wilson FC. Topical antibiotic irrigation in the prophylaxis of operative wound infections in orthopaedic surgery. Orthop Clin North Am. 1991;22(3):419-26.
25. Anglen JO. Comparison of soap and antibiotic solutions for irrigation of lower-limb open fracture wounds. A prospective, randomized study. J Bone Joint Surg Am. 2005;87(7):1415-22.
26. Demeulemeester E, Beliën J. Operating room planning and scheduling: a literature review. Eur J Oper Res. 2010;201(3): 921-32.
27. Parvizi J, Gehrke T. Proceedings of the International consensus meeting on periprosthetic joint infection. Bone joint J. 2013;90.

Postoperative Management

*Chetan Oswal, Sachin Jain,
Steve Rocha, Ashok Shyam, Anil Jain*

INTRODUCTION

Sophisticated prevention strategies have been developed during the past two decades to lower the risk of infectious complications in orthopedic surgeries. However, there is no proper consensus or guidelines regarding management of postoperative infection. Orthopedic surgeons are still in a dilemma about appropriate antibiotic prophylaxis and regarding the treatment also. Moreover, diagnosis and management require close collaboration between surgeons, infectious diseases specialists, microbiologists and pathologists, as no well-defined internationally accepted criteria for diagnosis and simultaneous treatment of orthopedic infections have been developed. We present appropriate guidelines related to the surgical wound and infection management in the postoperative period.

What is the optimal dressing material for a wound after the surgery?

The optimal dressing material should be low adherent, transparent polyurethane dressing, which protects the wound and gives the opportunity to check the surgical incision site for any signs of wound infection. Silver-impregnated dressings have not been conclusively shown to reduce surgical site infections (SSIs). Topical antimicrobial agents should not be used for wound dressing after surgery.

Explanation

It is generally considered best practice to cover all surgical incisions postprocedure with a low adherence, transparent polyurethane dressings, which protect the wound and give the opportunity to check the surgical incision site for any signs of wound infection without disturbing the dressing itself.[1] The advantages of using low adherent, transparent polyurethane film dressings in general are as follows:

- They allow postoperative inspection of the wound without disturbance of the dressing.
- They make the wound 'waterproof' to allow early showering or bathing, while at the same time acting both—a barrier to possible external bacterial contamination and to prevent cross contamination to other patients.
- Their low adherence allows relatively painless and easy removal when there is a need for a dressing change, such as when there is a build-up and leakage of exudates (oozing) from the incision site.
- They prevent any material from further contaminating the wound.
- They maintain an optimal moist wound environment without causing maceration of the surrounding skin, as the dressing material is permeable to moisture and gas.
- They prevent heat loss from the wound and maintain the optimal wound temperature.
- They provide a cost-effective approach to the wound management, as they reduce the number of dressing changes required and the pain experienced by the patient.

However, the Cochrane review study for the dressings for SSI in 2011 stated that there is no evidence to suggest that covering surgical wounds healing by primary intention with wound dressings reduces the risk of SSI or that any particular wound dressing is more effective than others in reducing the rates of SSI, improving scarring, pain control, patient acceptability or ease of dressing removal.[2] Hence, based on the current evidence, they concluded that decisions on wound dressing should be based on dressing costs and the symptom management properties offered by each dressing type.

Silver, as an antimicrobial agent, is particularly preferred, as it has a broad spectrum of antimicrobial activity with minimal toxicity toward mammalian cells at lower concentrations and has a less tendency than antibiotics to induce resistance due to its activity at multiple bacterial target sites.[3] However, silver-impregnated dressings have not been conclusively shown to reduce SSI. Trial et al.[4] conducted a randomized controlled trials (RCTs) where they compared silver-impregnated colloid dressings to non-silver dressings in treatment of variety of wound types including acute surgical wounds, infected and non-infected diabetic foot ulcers, and traumatic wounds. The above RCT failed to show any difference in terms of outcome in wound or ulcer healing and local infection rates. Hence, silver-impregnated dressings should not be used for routine, clean postoperative wound dressings. They are generally used as 'advanced dressings', where the wound is difficult to heal, such as chronic ulcers and burn wounds.[5]

Topical antimicrobial agents should not be used for surgical wounds that are healing by primary intention. Application of topical agents after surgery increases the risk of SSI.[1]

When is the first check dressing done after surgery and how often should it be done in postoperative period?

First check dressing should be done 48 hours after surgery or prior to discharging the patient from the hospital whichever is later. After that, the dressing in postoperative period should be done only if the dressing is soaked or then at the time of stitch removal.

> **Explanation**

The first check dressing is done 48 hours after surgery, as the surgical dressings are generally soaked in immediate postoperative period due to small exudates or discharge from the drain or the incision site. After that, in case of clean surgical cases, it is done only if the dressing has been soaked again. However, for open/compound wound, daily dressing is required.

Hence, the frequency at which the dressings are changed should be determined individually and will depend on the type of surgery, on the kind of wound dressing used and on host factors of the patient.[6]

What is the protocol for drain management in postoperative period?

For routine orthopedic surgeries, wound drains if kept should be removed after 24 hours after surgery or if the drain volume is less than 50 mL in the preceding 24 hours.

> **Explanation**

Closed suction drains reduce postoperative hematoma formation, but create an entry portal for bacteria and thus increase the risk of infection.[7] Drinkwater et al.[8] conducted a prospective clinical trial where wound drains were used in all patients having a total knee or total hip arthroplasty. Timing of drain removal and amount drained were recorded, and drain site swabs were sent with drain tips for bacteriology. The results of the above trial suggested that the likelihood of bacterial colonization increases, while wound drainage decreases with time. The authors concluded that the optimal time to remove drains is 24 hours after total joint arthroplasty.

However, a Cochrane review in 2011 about the use of surgical drains in orthopedic surgeries concluded that there is insufficient evidence from randomized trials to support or refute the routine use of closed suction drainage in orthopedic surgery and further randomized trials are required before definite conclusions can be made.[9] They pooled the results of various studies and indicated that there is no statistically significant difference in the incidence of wound infection, hematoma, dehiscence or reoperations between those allocated to drains and the undrained wounds.

Gaines et al.[10] also showed that there is no statistical difference in outcome between drained and undrained patients. The authors stated in orthopedics that, these devices have been used to decrease local edema, lessen the potential for hematoma or seroma formation, and to aid in the efflux of infection. However, the role of postoperative surgical drains in clean, elective cases has not been firmly established. Despite the paucity of clinical evidence demonstrating any benefit supporting their use, drains continue to be placed after elective orthopedic procedures.

Hence, we recommend that the timing of drain removal should be individualized according to the type of surgery. Drain can be removed after 24 hours for routine trauma, spine and arthroplasty cases. However, if large amount of drain volume is expected in such cases, drain should be removed, if the drain volume is less than 50 mL in the preceding 24 hours. For infected draining wounds also, the drain has to be kept for a longer time depending upon the amount of daily drainage.

What is the protocol for routine urinary catheterization in postoperative period?

Routine catheterization after orthopedic surgeries should be avoided. If at all urinary catheter is used, it can be kept for a maximum of 24–48 hours after surgery.

Explanation

Urinary catheters in the immediate postoperative period also acts as source of infection. Indwelling urinary catheters routinely in place for longer than 2 days postoperatively may result in excess nosocomial infections. Among patients with urinary tract infections (UTIs), an estimated 3.6% will develop bacteremia, a condition that adds significantly to hospital stay and is a risk factor for death among elderly patients.[11]

We do not recommend routine catheterization for most routine orthopedic surgeries. However, for prolonged surgeries of more than 2 hours, many surgeons do catheterize the patients. We recommend that the urinary catheter should be removed in the morning after the day of surgery for such mobile patients. For spine cases, it can be removed 48 hours postsurgery. For patients who are immobile and require longer catheterization period, a condom catheter or a silicon catheter should be used.

What is persistent wound drainage?

Persistent wound drainage is defined as continued drainage from the operative incision site for greater than 72 hours.

Explanation

Studies in the literature have a wide range of definitions for persistent wound drainage (48 hours to 1 week). However, limiting wound drainage to 72 hours postoperatively allows for earlier intervention and may limit the adverse consequences of persistent drainage.

Weiss and Krackow et al.[12] have defined[6] persistent wound drainage as fluid drainage occurring for 4 consecutive days beyond postoperative day 5; drainage that would significantly wet or soak at least a 2' × 2' area of gauze dressing and drainage that emanated from the same specific site (s) along the wound. Persistent wound drainage after surgery is also defined by time, type of secretion (hematogenous or clear), site (wound secretion, secretion after removal of suction drains) and microbial content. Simple spotting of dressings from poorly approximated wound edges, small areas of ulceration or marginal necrosis are not classified as persistent drainage.

For persistent wound drainage, how and when the wound culture should be done? What is the role of swabs?

Wound culture should be done in case of persistent wound drainage after 72 hours of surgery. In primary care, a swab is the most common method used for sampling a wound. Although biopsy or aspirates of pus are the 'gold standard' techniques, wound swabs can provide acceptable samples for bacterial culture, provided that the correct technique is used.

Explanation

Wound culture with the help of swabs is simple, inexpensive, non-invasive and convenient procedure for the majority of wounds. Swab sampling has been challenged on the basis that the superficial microbiology does not reflect that of deeper tissue and that subsequent cultures do not correlate with the presence of pathogenic bacteria. Also, if a swab sample is taken inappropriately (i.e. prior to wound cleansing and removal of devitalized superficial debris), the resulting culture has been considered to reflect only surface contamination and provide more false-negative results.[13]

If the wound is not purulent, it should be cleaned prior to swabbing. Some literature suggests that cleaning the wound before sampling is unnecessary; however, if the wound is not clean, it often leads to the isolation of multiple organisms, which may not be relevant and can generate laboratory results reporting 'mixed bacterial flora' rather than individual species. Cleaning removes the organisms present on the surface material, which are often different from those responsible for the pathology and allows for more accurate culture results. Wounds should be washed with sterile saline and then superficially debrided with a cotton-tipped swab.

Ideally, the patient should not have received recent antibiotic treatment before swabbing a wound, as this can affect the microbiological results.

The recommended swabbing procedure (Levine method)[14] are as follows:

- Apply sterile saline to moisten the head of the swab to increase the adherence of bacteria.
- Pass the swab over the wound area in a zigzag motion, while twisting the swab, so that the entire head of the swab comes into contact with the wound surface.
- Swab from the center of the wound outward to the edge of the wound.
- The swab should be pressed firmly enough that the fluid is expressed from the wound tissue (this may be painful for the patient).
- Repeat the process with a separate swab, if a pocket or sinus is present in the wound.

Swab culture is an important tool in the diagnosis of the infective organism. The Infectious Diseases Society of America (IDSA) guideline on the treatment of methicillin-resistant *Staphylococcus aureus* (MRSA) infections recommend obtaining cultures to guide systemic antibiotic therapy in purulent skin infections (e.g. associated with purulent drainage or exudates).[15]

Drinka et al.[16] in their study about swab cultures of purulent skin infection have stated that swabs should be used to determine if the wound is acutely infected and to identify potential pathogens in a wound that is judged to be infected based on clinical criteria. According to the authors, practitioners who utilize swab cultures to guide antibiotic selection for mild infections treated in the nursing home, should ensure proper collection technique and be aware that the results may indicate colonization rather than infection.

What are the pharmacological recommendations?

We recommend against administration of oral or intravenous (IV) antibiotics to patients with persistent wound drainage.

Explanation

Currently there is little to no evidence to support the administration of antibiotics to the patients with draining wound. Although the rationale for this practice appears logical, in that one is attempting to prevent ingress of infecting organisms through draining wound, the issue of emergence of antibiotic resistance and adverse effects associated with administration of antibiotics cannot be overlooked. In addition, administration of an antibiotic is likely to mask the underlying infection or make diagnosis of infection difficult by influencing the culture result.[17,18]

What is the protocol for anticoagulation in persistent draining wound and its effect on infection?

The decision about stoppage of anticoagulants should be based more on the clinical situation of the wound. These should generally be discontinued if there is persistent wound drainage for more than 48 hours. It is postulated that increased anticoagulation in a susceptible patient leads to increased wound soakage and consequently increased chances of infection.

Explanation

Generally, low molecular weight heparin (LMWH) is employed as a prophylactic agent for anticoagulation for most orthopedic surgeries. Advantages of LMWH over warfarin include its rapid onset of action and no need of monitoring after administration. However, its major adverse effect is increased risk of bleeding after administration. Monitoring of international normalized ratio (INR) value is also not beneficial, as LMWH does not affect it.[19]

Postoperative wound complications, including the development of hematoma and wound drainage are the significant risk factors for infection in the postoperative period. Increased anticoagulation will result more likely in the development of hematoma and wound drainage.

Hence, the decision to stop anticoagulant should be made on the wound status. In case of persistent wound drainage beyond 48 hours, it is advisable to stop anticoagulant.

There is very little evidence in literature on the recommendation of anticoagulation in case of persistent wound drainage. Parvizi et al[20] in his study about whether excess anticoagulation leads to periprosthetic infection have concluded that a mean INR of greater than 1.5 was found to be more prevalent in patients who developed postoperative wound complications and subsequent prosthetic joint infection (PJI), and hence cautious anticoagulation to prevent hematoma formation and/or wound drainage is critical to prevent PJI and its undesirable consequences. However, the therapeutic level of anticoagulation is the value of INR between 2 and 3. Hence, maintaining the value of INR below 1.5 serves no purpose of anticoagulation. We, thus, recommend that the INR value should be maintained below 2.5.

When should relook/debridement be done in persistent wound drainage?

A wound that has been persistently draining for more than 5 days should be operated upon without delay.

Explanation

Studies have shown that the risk of infection increase after 5 days of wound drainage. Thus, performing surgical intervention after 5 days is most appropriate for preventing the increased risk of SSI in the postoperative period.

The dilemma faced by the operative surgeon is when, if at all, to perform an irrigation and debridement for persistent

wound drainage. If such drainage is culture positive, then immediate intervention may clearly seem appropriate. However, in culture negative draining wounds, a balance must be sought between:
- Early irrigation and debridement, where a certain percentage of procedures would not, in retrospect, be found to have been necessary.
- Delay of operative treatment, which might lead to frank deep infection of the prosthesis in a percentage of cases.
- The possibility of introducing infection with an additional operative procedure.[21]

Drainage from the incision or from the drain site in the first few days after surgery can be managed with immobilization and sterile dressing changes. A strategy of immobilization and observation should not exceed 3–5 days.[22] Waiting for 5 days for the wound to dry may be secondary to anticoagulation use; therefore holding off the surgical intervention until postoperative day 5 is reasonable.

What are the modalities of investigation in a discharging wound?

Serum erythrocyte sedimentation rate (ESR), C-reactive protein (CRP) and white blood cells (WBCs) count are commonly used serological parameters, which are relatively non-specific markers.

Synovial fluid/aspirate analysis by arthrocentesis should also be employed in case of suspected prosthetic joint infection, if no overt clinical signs are present. Isolation of the causative organism by wound culture is the gold standard for diagnosis of infection. Blood culture may also be employed in case hematogenous spread of infection is suspected from other sites.

Explanation

Serum ESR and CRP are known sensitive markers of infection with relatively poor specificity and can be influenced by other infectious and non-infectious inflammatory diseases, including extra-articular infection. The ESR and the CRP level normally rises rapidly after surgery, reaching peak levels, several days after the operation with the CRP level peaking slightly earlier than the ESR. In the absence of an inflammatory arthropathy or infection, the serum level of CRP usually returns to normal by about 3 weeks after the surgery. The combination of an elevated ESR and CRP with traditional thresholds has been shown to be a more accurate predictor of infection than isolated elevations of the ESR or CRP alone. The ESR and CRP levels should be serially monitored every 3 days, in case infection is suspected. A declining/increasing trend of their levels will help to prognosticate the infection status.

White blood cell count is also elevated with relative increase in the polymorphonuclear leukocytes (PMNs). Leukocytosis commonly accompanies infection and may serve as an early marker for a developing infection. Leukocytosis is defined as a WBC count more than 11.0 cells × 10⁶/μL. However, postoperative leukocytosis is common after surgery and represents a normal physiologic response. In the absence of abnormal clinical signs and symptoms, we believe postoperative leukocytosis does not warrant further workup for infection.[23]

Synovial Fluid Analysis

A diagnostic arthrocentesis should be performed in all patients with suspected acute prosthetic joint infection unless the diagnosis is evident clinically. Synovial fluid analysis should include a total cell count and differential leukocyte count, as well as culture for aerobic and anaerobic organisms.[24] The cut-offs used to indicate infection:
- Synovial WBCs count more than 10,000 cells/μL
- Synovial PMN percentage more than 90%.

Blood cultures for aerobic and anaerobic organisms should be done if fever is present, if there is acute onset of symptoms or if the patient has a suspected infection, or a concomitant pathogen, which will make the presence of a bloodstream infection more likely.[25]

Microbiologic Cultures

The reference standard for diagnosing infection is the isolation of the responsible pathogen. However, standard microbiological cultures are only moderately sensitive and specific for diagnosing infection. A very low inoculum, adherent bacteria and the formation of small colony variants of microorganisms may limit detection. In addition, concurrent treatment with antimicrobial agents before sampling can prevent growth in the laboratory. Three specimens should be sent to the laboratory for accurate interpretation of the results. The diagnosis of orthopedic infections is established when all three specimens demonstrate growth of the same microorganism and the patient has clinically suspected infection.[26]

Does hospital stay cause infection? What is the optimum stay for patient after surgery? What is the role of extended intensive care unit (ICU) stay causing infection?

Longer pre and postoperative hospital including ICU stay leads to increased chances of infection. There is no consensus or guidelines on the optimum stay after surgery.

Explanation

Longer hospital stay is an independent risk factor even after adjusting for age, previous medical comorbidities, wound problems and development of medical complications.

One may hypothesize that with a longer hospital stay, patients are more likely exposed to nosocomial and virulent organisms that could result in later infection. In fact, the large incidence of infection by resistant organisms may relate partly to this factor.[27]

In case of clean surgeries, patient can be discharged on the 3rd day postoperatively after performing the first check dressing 48 hours postsurgery. Arthroplasty and spine patients can be discharged 5 days after surgery.

Farrin et al.[27] in his study about postoperative factors causing SSI has stated that patients with MRSA were 'more likely to have been in ICU, to have received antibiotics for more than 24 hours after the operation, to have had drains in place for more than 24 hours after the operation, and to have had more than 3 days of hospitalization immediately after surgery'.

Graf et al.[28] in his study about infection control measures, has also shown that the well-known independent risk factor for SSI occurrence is caused because of prolonged stay by the patient within the hospital prior to surgery and this also increases the risk of subsequent SSI occurrence.

SUMMARY

Monitoring of surgical wound in the postoperative period is essential to look for early signs of postoperative wound infection and to manage it accordingly. The optimal dressing material should be a transparent polyurethane dressing, which protects the wound and gives the opportunity to check the surgical incision site for any signs of wound infection. Silver-impregnated dressings have not been conclusively shown to reduce SSI. Topical antimicrobial agents are also to be avoided for wound dressing after surgery. The first check dressing should be done 48 hours after surgery. After that, the dressing in postoperative period should be done only if the dressing is soaked. Drains, catheter and IV line should be removed with a strict aseptic non-touch technique. Drains should be removed after 24 hours and urinary catheter should be removed after 48 hours of major surgeries.

Persistent wound drainage is defined as continued drainage from the operative incision site for more than 72 hours. A wound that has been persistently draining for more than 5 days should be operated upon without delay. Serum ESR, CRP and WBC count are commonly used serological parameters, which are relatively non-specific markers. Synovial fluid analysis by arthrocentesis should also be employed in case of suspected prosthetic joint infection, if no overt clinical signs are present. Isolation of the causative organism by wound culture is the gold standard for diagnosis of infection.

Surgical debridement of the wound should be done in case of persistent wound drainage beyond postoperative day 5. We recommend against administration of oral or IV antibiotics to patients with persistent wound drainage. Anticoagulation should be stopped in case of persistent wound drainage beyond 48 hours. The IV antibiotics should be given for a period of 2 weeks followed by a period of 4 weeks of oral antibiotics or longer depending upon the status of infection.

REFERENCES

1. National Collaborating Centre for Women's and Children's Health (UK). Surgical Site Infection: Prevention and Treatment of Surgical Site Infection. London: RCOG Press; 2008.
2. Dumville JC, Walter CJ, Sharp CA, et al. Dressings for the prevention of surgical site infection. Cochrane Database Syst Rev. 2011;(7):CD003091.
3. David Parson, Philip G, Silver Antimicrobial Dressings in Wound Management: A Comparison of Antibacterial, Physical, and Chemical Characteristics. Wounds. 2005;17(8):222-32.
4. Trial, Darbas H, Lavigne JP, et al. Assessment of the antimicrobial effectiveness of a new silver alginate wound dressing: a RCT. J Wound Care. 2010;9(1):20-6.
5. Silver dressings–do they work? Drug Ther Bull. 2010;48(4):38-42.
6. Ritting AW, Leger R, O'Malley MP, et al. Duration of postoperative dressing after mini-open carpal tunnel release: a prospective, randomized trial. J Hand Surg Am. 2012;37(1):3-8.
7. National Clinical Guideline Centre (UK). Infection: Prevention and Control of Healthcare-associated Infections in Primary and Community Care. London: Royal College of Physicians; 2012.

8. Drinkwater CJ, Neil MJ, et al. Optimal timing of wound drain removal following total joint arthroplasty. J Arthroplasty. 1995;10(2):185-9.
9. Parker MJ, Livingstone V, Clifton R, et al. Closed suction surgical wound drainage after orthopaedic surgery. Cochrane Database Syst Rev. 2007;(3):CD001825.
10. Gaines RJ, Dunbar RP, The use of surgical drains in orthopedics. Orthopedics. 2008;31(7):702-5.
11. Wold HL, Ma A, Bratzler DW, et al. Indwelling urinary catheter use in the postoperative period. Analysis of the national surgical infection prevention project data. Arch Surg. 2008;143(6):551-7.
12. Weiss AP, Krackow KA. Persistent wound drainage after primary total knee arthroplasty. J Arthroplasty. 1993;8(3):285-9.
13. Bowler PG, Duerden BI, Armstrong DG. Wound microbiology and associated approaches to wound management. Clin Microbiol Rev. 2001;14(2):244-69.
14. Gardner SE, Frantz RA, Saltzman CL, et al. Diagnostic validity of three swab techniques for identifying chronic wound infection. Wound Repair Regen. 2006;14(5):548-57.
15. Catherine Liu C, Bayer A, Cosgrove SE. Clinical practice guidelines by the Infectious Diseases Society of America for the treatment of methicillin-resistant Staphylococcus aureus infections in adults and children. Clin Infect Dis. 2011; 52:e18ee55.
16. Drinka P, Bonham P, Christopher J. Swab culture of purulent skin infection to detect infection or colonization with antibiotic-resistant bacteria. J Am Med Dir Assoc. 2012;13(1):75-9.
17. Hansen E, Durinka JB, Costanzo JA, et al. Negative pressure wound therapy is associated with resolution of incisional drainage in most wounds after hip arthroplasty. Clin Orthop Relat Res. 2013;471(10):3230-6.
18. Lonner JH, Lotke PA. Aseptic complications after total knee arthroplasty. J Am Acad Orthop Surg. 1999;7(5):311-24.
19. Sheth NP, Lieberman JR, Della Valle CJ. DVT prophylaxis in total joint reconstruction. Orthop Clin N Am. 2014;41(2): 273-80.

20. Parvizi J, Ghanem E, Joshi A, et al. Does 'excessive' anticoagulation predispose to periprosthetic infection? J Arthroplasty. 2007; 22(6 Suppl 2):24-8.
21. Saleh K, Olson M, Resig S, et al. Predictors of wound infection in hip and knee joint replacement: results from a 20 year surveillance program. J Orthop Res. 2002;20(3):506-15.
22. Deirmengian GK, Zmistowski B, Jacovides C. Leukocytosis is common after total hip and knee arthroplasty. Clin Orthop Relat Res. 2011;469(11):3031-6.
23. Yi PH, Cross MB, Moric M. Diagnosis of infection in the early postoperative period after total hip arthroplasty. Clin Orthop Relat Res. 2014;472(2):424-9.
24. Osmon DR, Berbari EF, Berendt AR, et al. Diagnosis and management of prosthetic joint infection: clinical practice guidelines by the Infectious Diseases Society of America. Clin Infect Dis. 2013;56(1):e1-25.
25. Wildmer AF. New Developments in Diagnosis and Treatment of Infection in Orthopedic Implants. Clin Infect Dis. 2001; 33(Suppl 2):S94-106.
26. Pulido L, Ghanem E, Joshi A, et al. Periprosthetic joint infection: the incidence, timing and predisposing factors. Clin Orthop Relat Res. 2008;466(7):1710-5.
27. Manian FA, Meyer PL, Setzer J, et al. Surgical site infections associated with methicillin-resistant Staphylococcus aureus: do postoperative factors play a role? Clin Infect Dis. 2003;36(7): 863-8.
28. Gray K, Vonberg R. Measures for the Prevention of Surgical Site Infections. In: Kon K, Rai M (Eds). Microbiology for Surgical Infections. Diagnosis, Prognosis and Treatment, 1st edition. USA: Elsevier; 2004. pp. 3-11.

10

Prophylactic Antibiotics

Mayur P Kardile, Chetan Oswal, Ashok Shyam, Parag Sancheti

INTRODUCTION

Principles of prophylactic antibiotic administration have proved to be a boon in surgical field. With the efficacy of prophylactic antibiotics in preventing surgical site infection (SSI), they have a high contribution in decreasing morbidity and making surgical procedures safe. Prophylactic antibiotic administration has proved to cut down infection rate in closed fractures from 5% to less than 1%.[1] However, there are still doubts regarding various issues like the appropriate antibiotic prophylaxis protocol, time and duration of administration. This chapter aims at giving comprehensive answers to these queries. With the rising prevalence of methicillin-resistant *Staphylococcus aureus* (MRSA) in perioperative infection, this chapter also discusses about MRSA screening and preoperative prophylaxis for the same. However, the duration of antibiotic holiday is not clear. The relevance of such antibiotic holiday has been discussed in this chapter. This chapter also addresses the issue pertaining to antibiotic allergies and provides a guideline for alternative antibiotic prophylaxis.

What is perioperative antibiotic protocol for closed and open fracture?

Closed fracture

For close fractures/clean elective surgeries use cefuroxime 1.5 g or cefazolin 2 g for three to five doses. First dose given

45–60 minutes before incision (additional dose should be given if surgical time exceeds 120 minutes) and other two or four doses spaced 12 hours apart over the next 1–2 days. For patients with MRSA colonization, vancomycin can be used as prophylaxis, which is to be started 120 minutes before incision and follow-up doses continued for 1–2 days more.

Explanation

There is a role of prophylactic antibiotics in managing open and closed fractures, and there is sufficient evidence that perioperative antibiotics decrease the risk of SSIs.[2–4] For closed fractures, cefuroxime, a second generation cephalosporin is given 1 hour before incision and should be continued for 24 hours after surgery. There is no evidence that continuing prophylactic antibiotics for a further period has any benefits.[2,5] Vancomycin can be used as prophylaxis for patients with MRSA colonization or in facilities with recent MRSA outbreaks:[2]

- Additional intraoperative doses of antibiotic are advised if:
  - The duration of the procedure exceeds one to two times the antibiotic's half-life
  - There is significant blood loss during the procedure.[6–8]
- The general guidelines for frequency of intraoperative administration are as follows (Table 10.1).[9]

Table 10.1: Frequency of antibiotics administration

Antibiotic	Frequency of administration
Cefazolin	Every 2–5 hour
Cefuroxime	Every 3–4 hour
Clindamycin	Every 3–6 hour
Vancomycin	Every 6–12 hour

Open Fractures

We recommend use of first generation cephalosporin + aminoglycoside + metronidazole for open fractures. Penicillin

20 lakh IU 4 hourly is given in case of barnyard injuries. For open fractures, antibiotics should be given at the time of arrival in casualty. Antibiotics should be given for 24 hours and for 24 hours after every subsequent debridement. No evidence to suggest the use of prophylactic antibiotics for a longer period.[10,11] Later antibiotics should be changed as per postdebridement culture reports.

Explanation

Antibiotics for open fractures,[12] according to Gustilo-Anderson classification system.

Table 10.2: Gustilo-Anderson classification system for antibiotics

Grades	Dosage
Grade I	First generation cephalosporin, cefazolin 2 g at every 8 hourly
Grade II	First generation cephalosporin, cefazolin 2 g at every 8 hourly
Grade III	First generation cephalosporin plus aminoglycoside, commonly gentamycin 3–5 mg/kg/day If barnyard injury, penicillin can be added, penicillin 20 lakh IU intravenously at 4 hourly If allergic to penicillin then vancomycin and clindamycin can be used

However, in our country with frequent presence of animal excreta on the roads, all patients should be given cephalosporin + aminoglycoside + metronidazole as prophylaxis.

Is there any role of switchover to oral antibiotics as prophylaxis after surgery?

All prophylactic antibiotics should be discontinued 24 to 48 hours postsurgery. There is no role of switchover therapy to oral antibiotics as prophylaxis.

Explanation

There is no evidence that continuing prophylactic antibiotics for a further period has any benefits.[2,10,11,13] Continuing antibiotics for more than that time may itself promote development of antibiotic resistance.[1]

How to choose an effective prophylactic antibiotic pertaining to a particular surgical site?

For all bone and joint surgeries, first and second generation cephalosporins are suitable antibiotics for prophylaxis.

Explanation

First and second generation cephalosporins are ideal for prophylaxis in all orthopedics surgeries.[14] They have a broad spectrum of action, cost effective and reserve more costly preparations for resistant organisms. They cover gram-positive organisms and also clinically important aerobic gram-negative and anaerobic gram-positive organisms.[7] They also have excellent distribution in synovium, muscle and hematoma;[15] they also achieve minimum inhibitory concentration (MIC) values rapidly after injection.[16–18]

What are the screening protocols for MRSA carriers?

Screening for MRSA is done for the staff at the time of joining the hospital. We may not regularly screen the patients for MRSA. Only patients transferred from other hospitals especially intensive care setups are screened for MRSA colonization.

What is the role of perioperative nasal mupirocin and shower wash or bath in known MRSA carriers?

Perioperative nasal mupirocin and shower wash or bath with 2% triclosan has been proved to significantly reduce the incidence of MRSA surgical site infections by reducing nasal carriage in endemic settings. However, this mupirocin use and shower wash with triclosan should only be given in patients who have been proven to be carriers of MRSA. Using this method as an empirical therapy fosters the growth of resistance organisms.

Explanation

In a controlled trial before and after approach in orthopedic wards, undergoing orthopedic surgery involving insertion of metal prosthesis and/or fixation, received perioperative prophylaxis with nasal mupirocin for 5 days and a shower wash or bath with 2% (v/v) triclosan before surgery [perioperative prophylaxis with nasal mupirocin treatment (PPNMT)]. After introduction of PPNMT there was a marked decrease in incidence of MRSA SSIs (per 1,000 operations) from 23 in the 6 months beforehand (period A) to 3.3 [($P < 0.001$), P stands for probability value] and 4 ($P < 0.001$) in subsequent consecutive 6-month periods (B and C respectively). Of 11 MRSA SSI cases that occurred during periods B and C, only one had actually received PPNMT, and 10 occurred after acute, as opposed to elective surgery ($P < 0.001$). Point prevalence nasal MRSA carriage decreased from 38% before PPNMT to 23% immediately after and 20%, 7%, 10% and 8% ($P < 0.001$) at 6-monthly intervals postintervention. This approach reduced the need of vancomycin usage by 23% and also there was no selection of mupirocin resistance in those patients.[19]

What is the ideal time for antibiotic with respect to tourniquet inflation?

Preoperative dose of antibiotic should be administered within 1 hour of tourniquet inflation. This time can be extended up to 2 hours for vancomycin and fluoroquinolones.

Explanation

The goal of administering preoperative antibiotics is to achieve adequate tissue concentrations before incision. The antibiotics should exceed MIC values for the organisms, which are likely to be encountered.[14]

In patients where tourniquet is used, patients obtained therapeutic evils of antibiotic in bone by 5 minutes after injection; however, it takes 10 minutes to achieve adequate concentration in subcutaneous tissues. Therefore, antibiotics should be administered at least 10 minutes or more before inflation of tourniquet.[20]

However, a recent study suggest that administration of prophylactic antibiotics before examination and inflation of a lower extremity tourniquet does not give better results than administration of the antibiotic shortly after inflation of the tourniquet.[21]

How can we test for allergy for antibiotics?

Allergy to antibiotics is to be tested by injecting intravenous (IV) 3-4 mL of diluted antibiotic solution and monitoring for adverse reactions. This first dose of antibiotic should be given in the recovery 60 minutes before the incision, so that any adverse reactions to the drug can be managed. In patients showing adverse reaction to cephalosporin, vancomycin or clindamycin can be used as alternate antibiotics.

Explanation

Skin testing should be done only in case of use of benzathine penicillin. For all other antibiotics, 3-5 mL of prepared antibiotic solution diluted in 10 mL normal saline is to be injected IV over 2-3 minutes and patient is monitored for occurrence of adverse drug reaction for next 10 minutes (Sanford guide to antimicrobial therapy 2012). If there is no adverse reaction, the rest of the antibiotic can be safely given. If adverse reaction is seen, the antibiotic injection is stopped.

Which antibiotic should be used in case a patient is allergic to β-lactam antibiotics?

When patient is allergic to penicillin, vancomycin and clindamycin can be used as alternate antibiotics for prophylaxis.

Explanation

In case of non-anaphylactic reaction to penicillin, a second generation cephalosporin can be used safely as there is limited cross reactivity. Patients with documented IgE mediated anaphylactic response, cephalosporins with R1 side chain similar to penicillin should be avoided (cefaclor, cefadroxil, cefatrizine, cefprozil, cephalexin, cephradine). Cephalosporins with different side chains can be used.[14]

Vancomycin and clindamycin have been recommended in patients with known type 1 β-lactam hypersensitivity reaction. Clindamycin is preferred as it has good bioavailability and at 30 minutes after infusion, it has shown to exceed MIC for *S. aureus*.[21] In *S. aureus*, clinical studies implicate that vancomycin increases the risk of SSI. Therefore a second agent should be added (levofloxacin and moxifloxacin) with vancomycin.[22-24]

SUMMARY

1. First and second generation antibiotics are sufficient in both open and closed fractures with addition of aminoglycoside required in heavily contaminated farm injuries.
2. Antibiotics should be administered around 60–45 minutes before surgery so that minimum inhibitory concentration is achieved.
3. Allergy to antibiotics is to be tested by injecting IV 3–4 mL of diluted antibiotic solution about 60 minutes prior to incision with monitoring for adverse reactions.
4. Screening for MRSA is done for the staff at the time of joining the hospital. We may not regularly screen the patients for MRSA. Only patients transferred from other hospitals especially intensive care setups should be screened for MRSA colonization.
5. In cases with β-lactam resistance, clindamycin is preferred over vancomycin as it reaches MIC faster.

REFERENCES

1. Bodoky A, Neff U, Heberer M, et al. Antibiotic prophylaxis with two doses of cephalosporin in patients managed with

internal fixation for a fracture of the hip. J Bone Joint Surg Am. 1993;75(1):61-5.
2. Bodoky A, Neff U, Heberer M, et al. Preoperative assessment of at-risk patients in traumatology. Helv Chir Acta. 1989;56(1-2): 91-5.
3. Prokuski L. Prophylactic antibiotics in orthopaedic surgery. J Am Acad Orthop Surg. 2008;16(5):283-93.
4. Boxma H, Broekhuizen T, Patka P, et al. Randomised controlled trial of single-dose antibiotic prophylaxis in surgical treatment of closed fractures: the Dutch Trauma Trial. Lancet. 1996;347(9009):1133-7.
5. Paiement GD, Renaud E, Dagenais G, et al. Double-blind randomized prospective study of the efficacy of antibiotic prophylaxis for open reduction and internal fixation of closed ankle fractures. J Orthop Trauma. 1994;8(1):64-6.
6. Mathur P, Trikha V, Farooque K, et al. Implementation of a short course of prophylactic antibiotic treatment for prevention of postoperative infections in clean orthopaedic surgeries. Indian J Med Res. 2013;137(1):111-6.
7. Dellinger EP, Gross PA, Barrett TL, et al. Quality standard for antimicrobial prophylaxis in surgical procedures. Infectious Diseases Society of America. Clin Infect Dis. 1994;18(3):422-7.
8. Bratzler DW, Houck PM. Antimicrobial prophylaxis for surgery: an advisory statement from the National Surgical Infection Prevention Project. Clin Infect Dis. 2004;38(12):1706-15.
9. Gross PA, Barrett TL, Dellinger EP, et al. Quality standard for the treatment of bacteremia. Infectious Diseases Society of America. Clin Infect Dis. 1994;18(3):428-30.
10. ASHP Therapeutic Guidelines on Antimicrobial Prophylaxis in Surgery. American Society of Health-System Pharmacists. Am J Health Syst Pharm. 1999;56(18):1839-88.
11. Dellinger EP, Caplan ES, Weaver LD, et al. Duration of preventive antibiotic administration for open extremity fractures. Arch Surg. 1988;123(3):333-9.
12. Dunkel N, Pittet D, Tovmirzaeva L, et al. Short duration of antibiotic prophylaxis in open fractures does not enhance risk of subsequent infection. Bone Joint J. 2013;95-B(6):831-7.

13. Robert W, Bucholz, Charles M, et al. Rockwood and Green's Fractures in Adults, 7th edition. Philadelphia: Lippincott Williams and Wilkins; 2009. p. 289.
14. Mathur P, Trikha V, Farooque K, et al. Implementation of a short course of prophylactic antibiotic treatment for prevention of postoperative infections in clean orthopaedic surgeries. Indian J Med Res. 2013;137(1):111-6.
15. Parvizi J, Gehrke T, Chen AF. Proceedings of the International Consensus on Periprosthetic Joint Infection. Bone Joint J. 2013;95-B(11):1450-2.
16. Neu HC. Cephalosporin antibiotics as applied in surgery of bones and joints. Clin Orthop Relat Res. 1984;(190):50-64.
17. Oishi CS, Carrion WV, Hoaglund FT. Use of parenteral prophylactic antibiotics in clean orthopaedic surgery. A review of the literature. Clin Orthop Relat Res. 1993;(296):249-55.
18. Schurman DJ, Hirshman HP, Kajiyama G, et al. Cefazolin concentrations in bone and synovial fluid. J Bone Joint Surg Am. 1978;60(3):359-62.
19. Wilcox MH, Hall J, Pike H, et al. Use of perioperative mupirocin to prevent methicillin-resistant Staphylococcus aureus (MRSA) orthopaedic surgical site infections. J Hosp Infect. 2003;54(3):196-201.
20. Zimmerli W. Infection and musculoskeletal conditions: Prosthetic-joint-associated infections. Best Pract Res Clin Rheumatol. 2006;20(6):1045-63.
21. Akinyoola AL, Adegbehingbe OO, Odunsi A. Timing of antibiotic prophylaxis in tourniquet surgery. J Foot Ankle Surg. 2011;50(4):374-6.
22. Hawn MT, Richman JS, Vick CC, et al. Timing of surgical antibiotic prophylaxis and the risk of surgical site infection. JAMA Surg. 2013;148(7):649-57.
23. Tetreault MW, Wetters NG, Aggarwal V, et al. The Chitranjan Ranawat Award: Should prophylactic antibiotics be withheld before revision surgery to obtain appropriate cultures? Clin Orthop Relat Res. 2014;472(1):52-6.
24. Johnson DP. Antibiotic prophylaxis with cefuroxime in arthroplasty of the knee. J Bone Joint Surg Br. 1987;69(5):787-9.

Further Reading

FURTHER READING

Although a lot of literature is available on the topics discussed in this book, we would like to suggest following to our readers for a more comprehensive read on the topics.

MAIN REFERENCES

1. Parvizi J, Gehrke T. Proceedings of the International Consensus on Periprosthetic Joint Infection. DTP publishing company; 2013.
2. Rutala WA, Weber DJ, Healthcare Infection Control Practices Advisory Committee (HICPAC). (2008). CDC-Guidelines for disinfection and sterilization in healthcare facilities. [online] Available from http://www.cdc.gov/hicpac/Disinfection_sterilization/toc.html [Accessed September 2014].
3. Harrop JS, Styliaras JC, Ooi YC, et al. Contributing factors to surgical site infections. J Am Acad Orthop Surg. 2012;20(2):94-101.
4. Recommended practices for sterilization. Perioperative Standards and Recommended Practices. Denver, CO: AORN, Inc: 2013. pp. 513-40.

BELOW ARE FURTHER READING FOR INDIVIDUAL CHAPTERS
SECTION 1: OPERATION THEATER NORMS AND PROTOCOLS

Chapter 1: Sterilization

1. Rutala WA, Weber DJ, Healthcare Infection Control Practices Advisory Committee (HICPAC). (2008). CDC-Guidelines for disinfection and sterilization in healthcare facilities. [online] Available from http://www.cdc.gov/hicpac/Disinfection_sterilization/toc.html [Accessed September 2014].
2. Recommended practices for sterilization. Perioperative Standards and Recommended Practices. Denver, CO: AORN, Inc: 2013. pp. 513-40.

Chapter 2: Operation Theater Planning and Protocols

1. Gupta SK, Kant S, Chandrashekhar R. Operating unit—planning essentials and design considerations. Journal of Academy of Hospital Administration. 2005;17:01-12.
2. Harsoor SS, Bhaskar SB. Designing an ideal operating room complex. Indian J Anaesth. 2007;51:193-9.
3. Worley DJ, Hohler SE. OR construction project: from planning to execution. AORN J. 2008;88(6):917-9, 923-34, 937-41.

Chapter 3: Surgeon Preparation and Scrubbing Protocols

1. WHO Guidelines on Hand Hygiene in Health Care: First Global Patient Safety Challenge Clean Care Is Safer Care; 2009.
2. AST Standards of Practice for Surgical Attire, Surgical Scrub, Hand Hygiene and Hand Washing. [online] Available from http://www.ast.org/uploaded Files/Main_Site/Content/About_Us/Standard_Surgical_Attire_Surgical_Scrub.pdf

Chapter 4: Laminar Airflow and Air-handling Unit

1. Thiele RH, Huffmyer JL, Nemergut EC. The "six sigma approach" to the operating room environment and infection. Best Pract Res Clin Anaesthesiol. 2008;22(3): 537-52.
2. Humphreys H, Taylor EW. Operating theatre ventilation standards and the risk of postoperative infection. J Hosp Infect. 2002;50(2):85-90.
3. Spagnolo AM, Ottria G, Amicizia D, et al. Operating theatre quality and prevention of surgical site infections. J Prev Med Hyg. 2013;54(3):131-7.

Chapter 5: Operation Theater Personnel

1. Centers for disease control and prevention. (2007). Guidelines for isolation precautions: preventing translation of infectious agents in healthcare settings. [online] Available from http://www.cdc.gov hicpac/2007ip_table.html [Accessed June 2014].
2. Allo MD, Tedesco M. Operating room management: operative suite considerations, infection control. Surg Clin North Am. 2005;85(6):1291-7.

SECTION 2: PERIOPERATIVE PATIENT PREPARATION

Chapter 6: Patient Optimization

1. Stryker LS, Abdel MP, Morrey ME, et al. Elevated postoperative blood glucose and preoperative hemoglobin A1C are associated with increased wound complications following total joint arthroplasty. J Bone Joint Surg Am. 2013;95(9):808-14, S1-2.
2. Olsen MA, Nepple JJ, Riew KD, et al. Risk factors for surgical site infection following orthopaedic spinal operations. J Bone Joint Surg Am. 2008;90(1):62-9.

Chapter 7: Patient and Operative Site Preparation

1. Reichman DE, Greenberg JA. Reducing surgical site infections: a review. Rev Obstet Gynecol. 2009,2(4): 212–21.
2. Drosou A, Falabella A, Kirsner RS. Antiseptics on Wounds: An Area of Controversy. Wounds. 2003;15(5):799-801.

Chapter 8: Intraoperative Protocols

1. Yammine K, Harvey A. Efficacy of preparation solutions and cleansing techniques on contamination of the skin in foot and ankle surgery: A systematic review and meta-analysis. Bone Joint J. 2013;95-B(4):498-503.
2. Tejwani NC, Immerman I. Myths and legends in orthopaedic practice: are we all guilty? Clin Orthop Relat Res. 2008;466(11):2861-72.

Chapter 9: Postoperative Management

1. Anglen JO. Comparison of soap and antibiotic solutions for irrigation of lower-limb open fracture wounds. A prospective, randomized study. J Bone Joint Surg Am. 2005;87(7):1415-22.
2. Dressings for the prevention of surgical site infection. Cochrane Review 2011.
3. Karolin Graf and Ralf-Peter Vonberg. Infection control measures for the prevention of surgical site infections. In: Kateryna Kon, Mahendra Rai (Eds). Microbiology for Surgical Infections: Diagnosis, Prognosis and Treatment. Academic Press; 2014. pp. 1-54.

Chapter 10: Prophylactic Antibiotics

1. Prokuski L. Prophylactic antibiotics in orthopaedic surgery. J Am Acad Orthop Surg. 2008;16(5):283-93.
2. Dunkel N, Pittet D, Tovmirzaeva L, et al. Short duration of antibiotic prophylaxis in open fractures does not enhance risk of subsequent infection. Bone Joint J. 2013;95-B(6):831-7.